Skin Microbiome

Your Invisible Whispers

Dr Karnika Saigal,
Dr Kashish Kalra

notionpress.com
INDIA • SINGAPORE • MALAYSIA

ISBN

Paperback ISBN: 979-8-90269-557-8

Hardcase ISBN: 979-8-90269-558-5

Contents

About the Authors

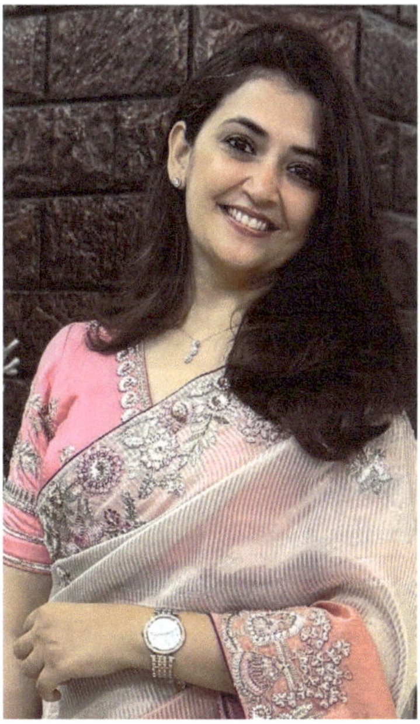

Dr. Karnika Saigal, is a medical microbiologist with a deep interest in human microbial infections and their impact on health. She earned her M.B.B.S. and M.D. in Microbiology from the Postgraduate Institute of Medical Sciences, Chandigarh, and has served as a medical microbiologist at the Dr. R.P. Centre, All India Institute of Medical Sciences (AIIMS), New Delhi.

Following her fellowship in aesthetic medicine, Dr. Saigal's research began focusing on the intricate relationship between the skin barrier and the human microbiome. With over twelve years of experience in studying human–microbe interactions, her work explores the dynamic interface between skin health and microbial ecology.

Through her writing, she strives to bridge the gap between laboratory science and clinical dermatology—promoting evidence-based skincare and microbiome-conscious therapeutics for a healthier, balanced skin ecosystem.

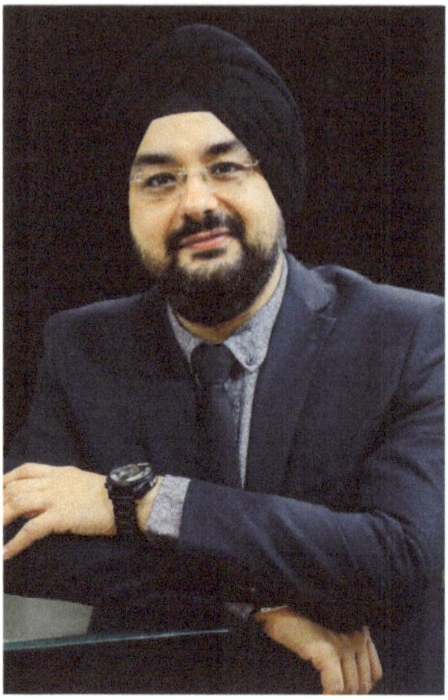

Dr. Kashish Kalra, is a board-certified Dermatologist recognized by the Delhi Medical Council and the Medical Council of India. He completed his MD in Dermatology from Sarojini Naidu Medical College, Agra and trained extensively at Dr. P.N. Behl's Skin Institute & School of Dermatology, New Delhi.

Currently serving as Head of the Department of Dermatology and Trichology at Max Smart Hospital, Saket, and as Director of Dr. Kalra's Skin Clinic, Jangpura Extension, New Delhi, he combines clinical expertise with a passion for research.

Dr. Kalra's work explores the intersection of dermatology, microbiology, and barrier science, with a special focus on how the skin microbiome influences health, disease, and aesthetic outcomes. Trained internationally under the European Academy of Dermatology and Venereology and at Toulouse, France, he continues to advance evidence-based dermatology through innovation, education, and compassionate care.

Foreword

Beneath the surface lies a bustling world of bacteria, fungi, and viruses, shaping your skin's beauty and resilience. Explore the science of skin and gut communication, and learn how nurturing this ecosystem transforms your health.

Chapter Summary

Chapter 1: Healthy Skin – Factors Influencing My Happy Home

- Introduction to skin microbiome
- Skin as an ecosystem: structure and functions
- Microbial residents: bacteria, fungi, viruses, and mites
- Role of microbiome in skin health
- Endogenous vs. environmental factors
- Resident vs. transient microbes
- Life in a microbial city: biofilms, quorum sensing, microbial families
- Delicate balance and dysbiosis
- **Key Takeaways**

Chapter 2: Age and Skin Microbiota – The Aging Skin Microbiome

- Microbial evolution from birth to old age
- Infant skin colonization and microbial inheritance
- Puberty: hormonal changes and microbial shifts
- Adulthood and microbial stability

Acknowledgement

To the invisible guardians that live on and within us, teaching us balance and resilience—thank you.

To our family, friends, and mentors, whose love, guidance, and curiosity lit the way—this journey is yours as much as ours.

A special thanks to the invisible guide-AI tools for book editing and transforming science into stories.

May this book be a tribute to the quiet worlds that shape us, and an invitation to see the beauty in what we cannot always see.

Special thanks

“To our parents, whose quiet strength and boundless love have lifted us through every challenge and celebrated every joy.”

“To our daughters, Kashika and Kairaa, thank you for filling life with wonder, curiosity, and laughter you make every discovery brighter.

Chapter 1

Healthy Skin

Factors influencing my happy home

You may not know me well, but I've been with you since the moment you were born. I am your **skin microbiome**—the invisible community that calls your skin home. You can't see me, but I'm always here, quietly working to keep your skin balanced, resilient, and alive.

Your skin—my home— is the body's largest organ, covering 1.5 to 2 square meters (15 to 20 square feet) of surface area of a human body.

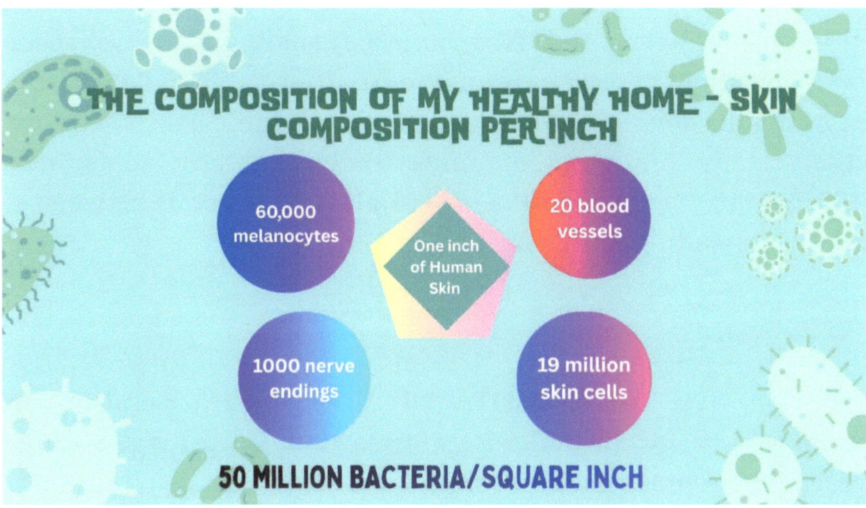

Before I tell you more about myself, let me share why your skin is extraordinary:

1. It is your **first line of defence**, keeping harmful invaders out.
2. It gives you **sensation**—heat, cold, touch, even pain.
3. It helps regulate your **temperature**, keeping you comfortable.
4. It reflects your **emotions**—blushing, sweating, goosebumps.

- Your **armpits and groin** are warm and humid, like tropical rainforests.
- Your **hands and feet** are drier, more like deserts.
- Wherever oil glands cluster, special microbes thrive in abundance

Imagine your skin as a vast, living landscape: rolling hills and valleys, rivers of sweat, forests of hair, and oil-rich lakes called sebaceous glands. But here's the interesting part: not all areas of your skin are the same. Differences in skin topography are observed throughout your body; the location of the skin determines the regional topography of your skin. Temperature and humidity are higher at moist sites, such as the groin or armpit (approaching 37°C, the body's core temperature), and lower in the body's extremities (fingers and toes, approximately 30°C). **Sebaceous gland density of your skin is an important variable in determining the local microbial niche at the given site of skin.** Sebaceous glands secrete many lipidic compounds, including fatty acids; these contribute to the acidification of skin pH (which varies between 4.2 and 7.9 depending on the site).

Meet My Family

My home, THE **MICROBIOTA OF YOUR SKIN,** points to the assemblage of specific microorganisms that are present within a defined environment. Interestingly, your skin is home to millions of us, including bacteria, fungi, viruses and mites (*Demodex).*

We may not be as famous as your gut microbes, but we are your body's **second largest microbial community**. In fact, every square centimetre of your skin can host anywhere from **10,000 to 1,000,000** of us. Scientists have identified more than **200 genera** living here!

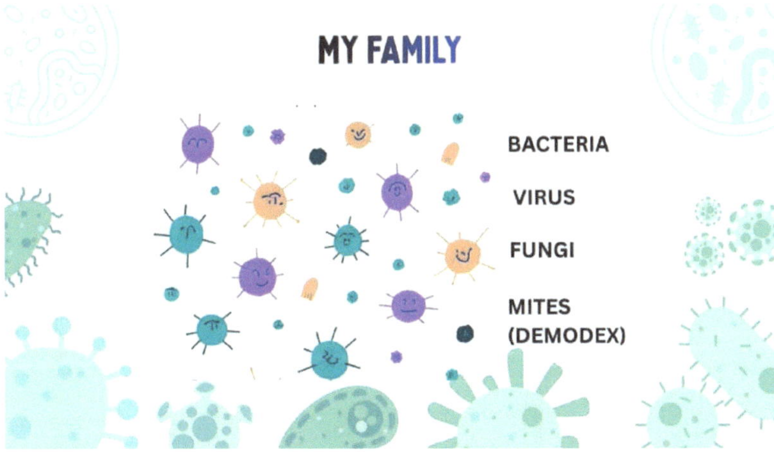

You might wonder, why should you care about me? Here's why:

My healthy home, the microbiome, provides a multitude of benefits to the host body:

My key role in maintaining healthy skin is to regulate homeostasis.

- I **protect your skin** by occupying space and resources so harmful microbes can't take over.
- I **produce nutrients** such as vitamins and amino acids.
- I **train your immune system**, keeping it alert but not overreactive.
- I **support skin renewal**, helping cells stay active and healthy.

Shaping of My World; Factors influencing my healthy home (skin microbiome):

My home—your skin—is shaped by forces both inside you and around you. Together, your skin topography, skin functions, and microbial composition are influenced by body site and a range of endogenous (e.g., genetics, age and gender) and environmental (e.g., lifestyle, climate, air pollution and use of cosmetics) factors.

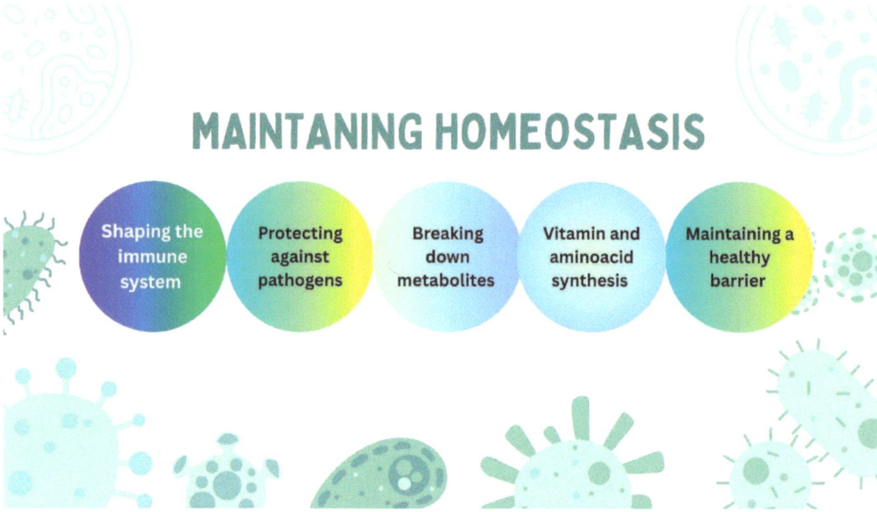

The vulnerability of my microbial network depends on many intrinsic and extrinsic factors that your skin is exposed to.

Your **age, genetics, ethnicity, climate, and skincare habits** all shape these microbial landscapes, making your skin's ecosystem unique to you.

A. Endogenous Factors: Being exposed to the external environment, your skin itself has strong defence mechanisms to protect you from harmful microbes.

- **Genetics, age, and gender** define my blueprint.
- Your **skin barrier** protects us both—
    - **Keratin** is the shield; it presents a tough physical barrier to most microorganisms. It makes the skin resistant to weak acids and bases, bacterial enzymes, and toxins
    - **Acidic pH (5.4–5.9)** deters invaders. The acidic environment of skin (pH of 5.4 to 5.9) also creates an inhospitable environment for potential pathogens and inhibits bacterial growth. Low skin pH also conserves the commensal skin microflora, which act as a first-line defence against pathogens through direct competition,

influencing cutaneous immunity and supporting barrier homeostasis.

- **Sebum** feeds me while blocking harmful microbes. Sebum produced by the sebaceous glands acts as a seal for hair follicles and contains several antimicrobial molecules as well as specific nutritional lipids for beneficial microorganisms.

- **Mucosae** in which my home resides: comprises a glycoprotein layer on top of the epithelium, housing the commensal microorganisms. The epithelial membranes produce protective chemicals that eliminate many microorganisms and maintain my healthy home.

LAYERS OF SKIN

Epidermis-

- largest epithelial surfaces for interaction with microbes
- Protective barriers
- Immune barrier
- Imparts Color (melanin pigment)
- Renews skin

Dermis –

- Ninety percent of skin's thickness
- Composed of collagen and elastin
- Keep skin resilient and flexible
- Encloses hair roots
- Produces oil/sebum
- Produce sweat via sweat glands
- Perceives sensations and pain with large network of nerves across,
- Supplies blood and nutrients

Hypodermis –

- Fatty layer.
- Cushions the muscles and bones
- Nerves and blood vessels in the dermis (middle layer) get larger in the hypodermis

(Photo credit: WebMD)

B. Environmental Factors:

- **Climate, pollution, lifestyle, pets, and even the people you live with** shape my community. Differences are observed in the skin microbiome of people living in different environmental conditions, including the influence of geographic location, occupation, and exposure to domestic animals. The skin microbiome of people who live together tends to show similarity, even if they are not genetically related or intimate with each other.

- **Cosmetic products** can either help me or disrupt my balance—your daily choices truly matter; they significantly affect the skin microbiota and thus should be used according to the skin type.

Extrinsic and Intrinsic Factors influencing Skin

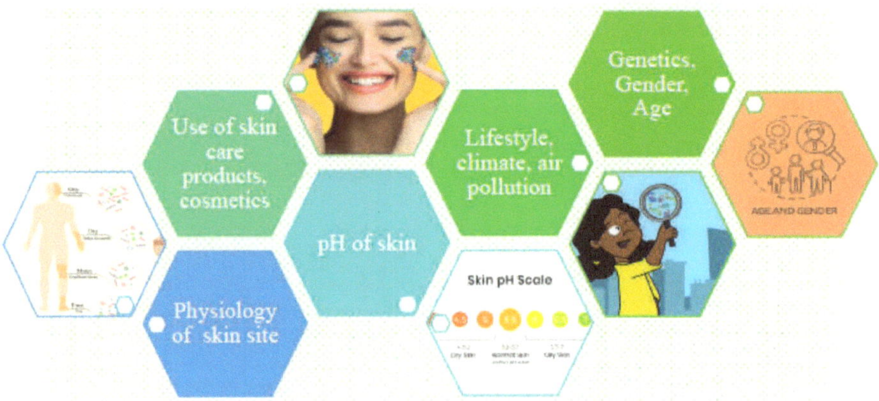
Use of skin care products, cosmetics
Genetics, Gender, Age
Lifestyle, climate, air pollution
pH of skin
Physiology of skin site
Skin pH Scale
AGE AND GENDER

Each human has a specific signature microbiome depending upon the intrinsic and extrinsic factors.

Skin vs. Gut Microbiome Survival

Life on the skin is far tougher than life in the gut. While gut microbes feast on a constant supply of dietary micro- and macronutrients, skin microbes must adapt to a limited diet of **proteins, lipids, sweat, and sebum**.

- The **stratum corneum**, the skin's outer layer, provides keratin and lipids.
- **Sweat glands** contribute water, salts, lactate, and urea.
- **Sebaceous glands** supply sebum, a nutrient-rich lipid mixture.

Skin microbiota are specialists, evolved to survive in environments that are:

- **Cooler and acidic** (pH ~5.4–5.9)
- **Dry or intermittently moist**
- **Variable in oxygen** (aerobic at surface, anaerobic in follicles)
- **Exposed to UV radiation**

These adaptations explain why microbes such as *Cutibacterium*, *Staphylococcus*, and *Malassezia* are able to colonize specific niches—oily, moist, or dry regions—while maintaining the delicate balance of a healthy skin microbiome.

Stability of Skin Microbial Niches

Even though your skin is constantly exposed to changing environments, its microbial communities are surprisingly stable over time. The composition of these communities depends largely on the **physiology of the site**—whether the area is sebaceous (oily), moist, or dry.

- **Sebaceous sites** (like the face and back) host the most stable communities, dominated by lipid-loving microbes such as *Cutibacterium acnes*.
- **Moist areas** (such as armpits and groin) favor *Staphylococcus spp.* and *Corynebacterium spp.*
- **Dry zones** (like forearms and palms) contain more mixed and variable microbes.
- **Feet** have the least stable microbiota, constantly influenced by footwear, sweat, and external contact.

The Residents and the Visitors

- **Resident flora (core microbiota):** Long-term stable species adapted to your skin (e.g., *Staphylococcus epidermidis*).
- **Transient flora:** Microbes acquired through contact with surfaces, people, or environment. Normally cleared quickly, but if your barrier weakens, they may colonize and cause infection.

Most of us are **loyal residents**, staying with you for life (residential flora). But there are also **transient microbes**—wanderers who arrive when you touch surfaces, meet people, or explore your surroundings. A large proportion of my family members form stable residential microbial niches throughout your skin. However, a small percentage of notorious members from my family are present transiently (called transient microbes) and can opportunistically make your skin their permanent residence if your skin health/your skin barrier is compromised. The tricky situation thus created, i.e., disruption of microbial balance between good and harmful microbes, can result in skin diseases.

Life in Our Microbial City

Think of us as a bustling city full of life and work to do. **The microbiota of your skin** is actually not just a small family but a group of families living in harmony within your skin. We have our well-protected, robust houses (biofilms), our own neighbourhood, and yes, we talk (quorum sensing).

Like humans, we also have kingdoms, families (phyla), specific familial names (genus), castes (species) and subcastes (subspecies/strains), each with different roles. Bacteria are the most abundant kingdom across sites, and fungi are among the least. Skin is home to 18 phyla (families) of the bacterial kingdom, with four predominant ones (names are tough, but we are unique in our own sense):

Actinobacteria, Firmicutes, Proteobacteria and Bacteroidetes. Depending upon the favourable conditions at each site of your skin, there is a relative abundance of particular families; we establish our colonies at specific sites.

- We build **biofilm houses** to stay safe.
- We **communicate using quorum sensing**, chemical "conversations" that help us coordinate.
- We **organize into families, species, and strains**, each with different roles.

To make our world understandable to humans, scientists have tried to observe our growth characteristics and our environmental behaviours, have decoded us through microscopes and have even employed an array of molecular tests for our genetic analysis.

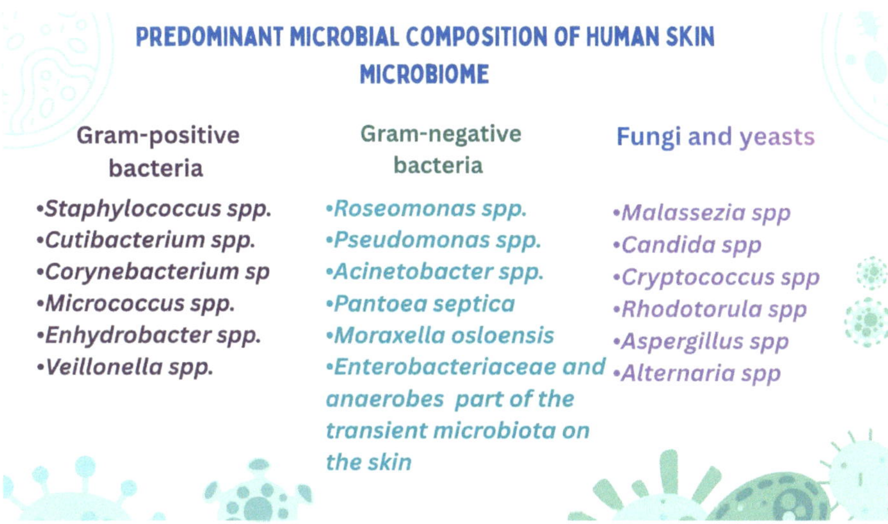

Who Lives Where on Your Skin?

Different regions of your skin host distinct microbial specialists, each adapted to the nutrients and conditions available: Microbes that lack the property to produce their own food (auxotroph) thrive on the lipids of sebum present in your skin.

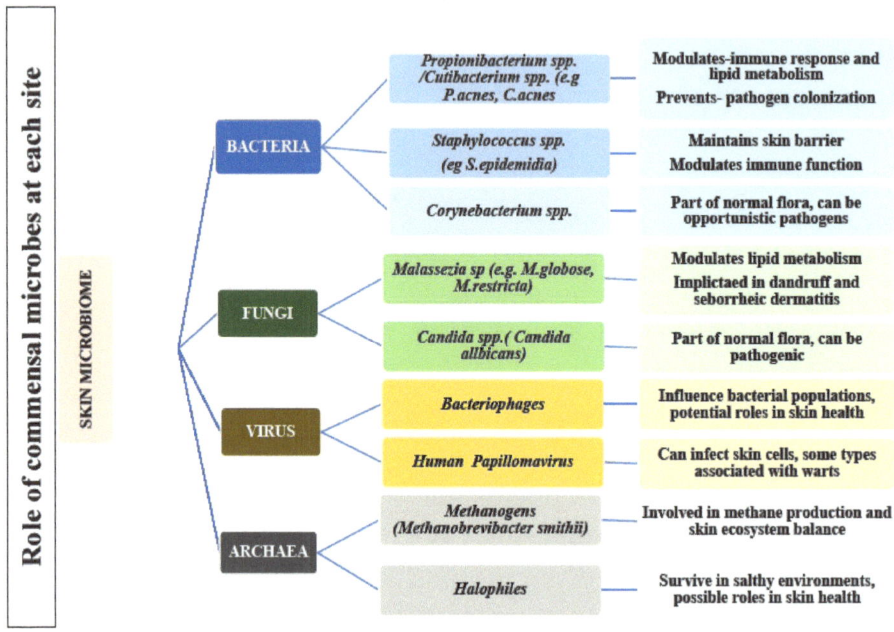

- **Sebaceous (oily) sites** – Rich in sebum, these areas are dominated by *Propionibacterium spp.* (now re-classified as *Cutibacterium spp.*), lipophilic bacteria that thrive in low-oxygen environments and are linked to acne.
- **Moist areas (elbows, feet, armpits)** – Nutrients like salts, sterols, esters, and lipids support commensals such as *Staphylococcus* and *Corynebacterium*. These bacteria have evolved survival strategies, including tolerance to sweat's high salt levels and the ability to use urea as a nutrient.
- **Fungal residents** – *Malassezia* species dominate across almost all body sites, maintaining skin homeostasis, with other genera like *Rhodotorula, Cryptococcus,* and *Candida* present in smaller numbers. Unlike bacteria, fungal colonization is relatively uniform across the skin.
- **Viruses** – Viral colonization tends to be highly individual, shaped more by the host than by the site on the body.
- **Mites** – Tiny arthropods such as *Demodex* inhabit seborrheic regions like the face (eyelids, nasal folds) and hair follicles.

Together, we microbes illustrate how skin is not a single environment but a mosaic of evolving niches—each selecting for residents uniquely adapted to survive there.

A Delicate Balance

We are simple; we were before you on earth and will remain even after you. We are omnipresent throughout your body; our presence in the correct amount labels your skin health. Overall, the skin harbours a heterogeneous community of microorganisms, and each microbe has distinct adaptations to survive on the skin. Microbes reside and form specific skin niches, with community structure linked to skin region and age-related changes.

> We have been here long before humans, and we'll be here long after. But our harmony is delicate.
>
> - When balance holds → your skin glows with health.
> - When balance breaks → dysbiosis occurs, leading to conditions like acne, dandruff, psoriasis, dermatitis, or even hair loss.

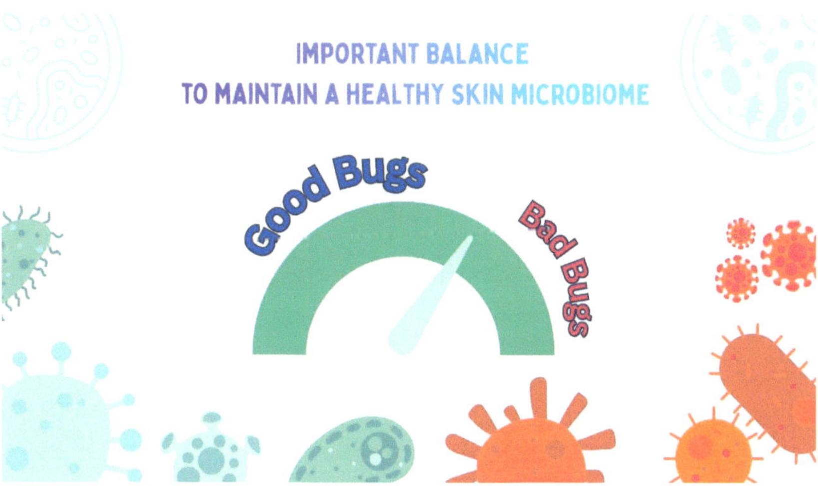

The microbial dysbiosis, i.e., the break in the balance of healthy skin microbiota, has been linked to various cutaneous diseases such as acne vulgaris, psoriasis, atopic dermatitis, rosacea, seborrheic dermatitis, dandruff, alopecia areata, impaired wound healing, and hidradenitis suppurativa.

My Promise to You

I am your invisible partner, always protecting and balancing your skin. Care for me—choose products wisely, nourish your body, live in balance—and I will continue to guard your skin's resilience. Because your healthy skin is not just your home—it is mine too.

Key Takeaways

Your skin is your **largest organ** and a diverse microbial landscape.

- The **skin microbiome** (bacteria, fungi, viruses, mites) protects, nourishes, and balances skin health.
- Both **internal factors** (genetics, age, natural defences) and **external factors** (environment, lifestyle, cosmetics) shape your microbiome.
- **Each human has a specific signature microbiome** depending on the intrinsic and extrinsic factors.
- Most microbes are **stable residents**, while some are **transient visitors** that may cause trouble if balance is lost.
- **Dysbiosis** leads to conditions like acne, dandruff, psoriasis, or dermatitis.
- On your skin, dominant families:
    - **Actinobacteria** (e.g., *Propionibacterium*) thrive in oily zones, sometimes linked to acne.
    - **Firmicutes** (e.g., *Staphylococcus*) and ***Corynebacterium*** prefer moist folds.

- **Fungi** like *Malassezia* are everywhere, usually peaceful neighbours.
- **Viruses** live more individually, tied to you rather than your environment.

Mites (*Demodex*), quietly living in your hair follicles.
"I am your skin's invisible companion, always at work to protect and balance you. Care for me, and together we will keep your skin healthy, strong, and glowing."

Chapter 2

Age and Skin Microbiota

The Ageing Skin microbiome

Age: a word that defines you're alive, is inevitable.

Ageing is a process that every living form undergoes. I grow with you. From the moment you were born, my family—the microbes on your skin—has evolved alongside you. Just as your body changes, so does your microbial world. Age is not just a number for humans; it is a signal for us, your skin microbiome, to adapt.

Your skin's physiology changes over time, influenced by **genetics, gender, environment** (pollution, sun exposure, and climate)**, and lifestyle** (exercise, stress, sleep, nutrition, and skincare routine). These factors shape not only your skin's appearance but also the microbial neighbourhoods I inhabit.

How Aging Shapes My Home

As you age, your skin undergoes many changes: significant alterations in the skin surface's physiology result in shaping site-specific microbial niches. Skin aging is characterized by a decrease in sebum, sweat, and immune function, resulting in significant alterations in the skin surface's physiology, including lipid composition, sebum secretion, and pH.

- **Sebum production decreases** → drier skin
- **Sweat gland activity declines** → reduced cooling and microbial hydration
- **Immune function weakens** → higher susceptibility to infections
- **pH shifts** → altered microbial niches

These changes affect **moisture, collagen, and elasticity**, creating new challenges for both skin and microbiome.

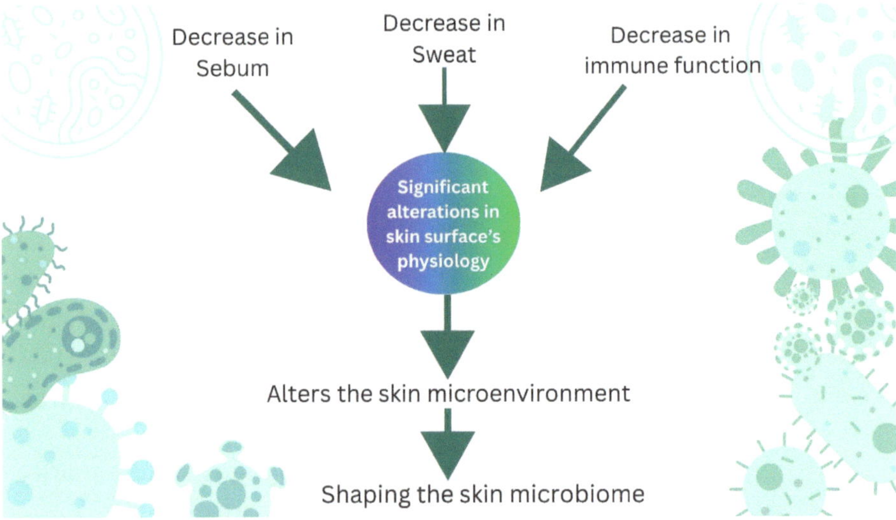

Unlike your gut microbiome, which stabilizes around age three, my skin population continues to shift throughout life. **Each stage—infancy, puberty, adulthood, old age—brings different skin microbial residents.** A naturally aged skin, featuring varied physiological and structural modifications, exhibits drastic compositional alterations in residential microbial niches throughout your skin. Healthy adults stably maintain the composition of their skin microbial communities for at least 2 to 4 years, assessed.

Skin Microbiome Across the Lifespan

- **Infant Skin**
  - Thinner, more alkaline, higher cell turnover.
  - Microbiota less diverse, dominated by *Staphylococcus spp.* and *Streptococcus spp.*
- **Puberty**
  - Surge in sebum production.
  - Oily niches expand, favoring *Cutibacterium spp.* (linked to acne).

- **Adulthood**
  - Microbial diversity stabilizes.
  - Balanced communities of *Staphylococcus spp*, *Corynebacterium spp*, *Cutibacterium spp*, and *Malassezia spp*.
- **Elderly Skin**
  - Reduced sebum and sweat.
  - Skin becomes drier, less acidic → shifts in microbial balance, higher susceptibility to infections.

"Skin Microbiome Dynamics Across the Human Lifespan"

The earliest encounters of your skin with me—right at birth—set the stage for the future. Early colonization not only seeds my communities but also helps train your developing immune system. My first contact with your skin is crucial for the development of infant immunity, favourably developing tolerance to skin commensals. This first dialogue between your skin and me builds tolerance to beneficial commensals while teaching your immune defences to stay alert against invaders. In this way, your skin microbiome in adulthood carries the imprint of its earliest microbial friendships. Healthy skin microbiome development in early life provides insight into the associations between microbial dysbiosis and pathology, making skin microbiota a crucial predictor of diseases in adulthood.

Infant Skin – My First Contact

Even before you are born, colonization may begin.

- **Vaginal birth:** you inherit microbes from your mother's vaginal canal (mainly *Lactobacillus spp*, *Prevotella spp*).
- **Caesarean birth:** skin-associated microbes of the mother or primary care givers dominate (e.g., *Staphylococcus spp*, *Corynebacterium spp*, *Cutibacterium spp*).

By six weeks, early differences fade, and by three months, **site-specific microbial patterns** emerge. By one year, diversity stabilizes.

Key facts of infant skin:

1. Colonization may start in utero.
2. Birth expands microbial exposure rapidly.
3. Delivery mode influences early microbiome.
4. Differences fade after 6 weeks.
5. Antibiotic exposure during pregnancy or birth can impact microbial balance.
6. Infant skin is **thinner, more alkaline**, and changes faster than adult skin.
7. Early microbial colonization lays the foundation for **immunity and resilience** later in life.

Puberty – A Microbial Revolution

The changing microenvironment of different skin sites during your sexual maturation influences my microbial niches, i.e., your skin microbiome. Hormones awaken during puberty, stimulating **sebaceous glands**. Oil-rich skin attracts microbes that thrive on lipids, including *Propionibacterium spp*, *Corynebacterium spp*, and *Malassezia spp*.

This shift explains why teenagers often experience acne and other skin changes—it's a visible sign of my evolving community.

Adulthood to Old Age – The Slow Transition

During adulthood, my microbial communities stabilize but remain **site-specific**. As age progresses:

- **Sebum decreases**, skin dries, pH shifts.
- **Immune function weakens**, making the barrier more fragile.
- **Skin aging accelerates**, with higher susceptibility to infection, irritation, and diseases.

Skin microbiome as we age:

1. *Staphylococcus epidermidis:* Still abundant but may decrease slightly in diversity and protective function.
2. *Cutibacterium (Propionibacterium) acnes:* Markedly decreases with age due to reduced sebum (oil) production.
3. *Corynebacterium spp.:* Increases relatively as sebaceous bacteria decline.
4. *Staphylococcus aureus:* May become more prevalent, especially on compromised or dry skin, contributing to inflammation or infection risk.
5. *Micrococcus luteus:* Often increases on aged skin; adapted to drier, oxygen-rich environments.
6. *Malassezia spp. (especially M. restricta and M. globosa):* Usually decrease with reduced lipid availability in older skin.
7. *Candida spp.:* May increase, especially in warm, moist, or immunocompromised areas.

The fact that microbial niches and the skin microbiome of young children and adults are different, likewise the skin care regimen and skin products of both the age groups differ. Thus, caution must be kept in mind while dealing with patients.

Major Microbial Changes as you age

- Reduced overall diversity in some skin sites.
- Shift from oily to dry-type microbes due to lower sebaceous activity.
- Delayed wound healing and altered immune-microbe signaling.

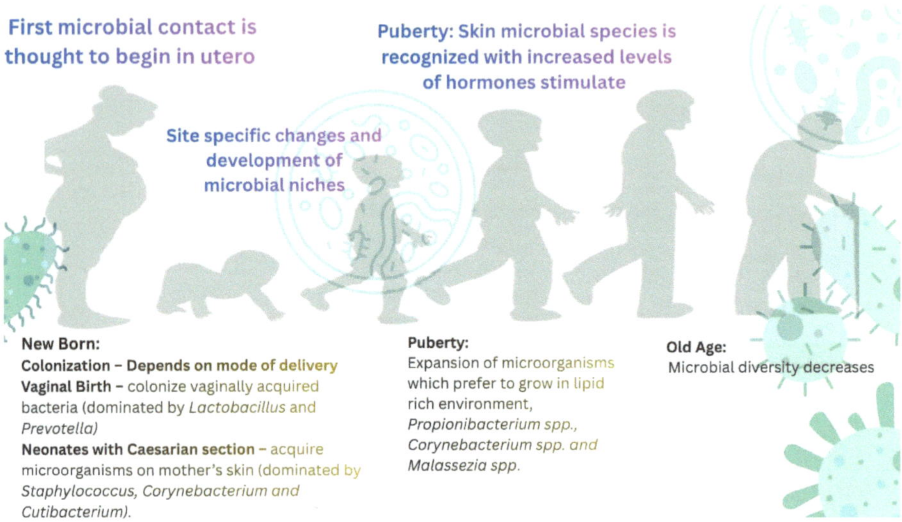

Even the **gut microbiome** changes with age, and this affects my home on your skin.

Gut–Skin Connection in Aging

You see, your gut is my distant cousin in a way. When it thrives, it sends out friends and allies that keep me balanced and happy. But when the gut falls into dysbiosis—a state where helpful microbes dwindle and harmful ones take over—it can create chaos.

As you journey from adulthood into old age, the changes in your skin microbiota are mirrored by equally profound shifts in your gut microbiome. Scientists now know that the gut microbial community does more than aid digestion—it plays a role in how quickly or gracefully you age. Within your gut live specialized bacteria that produce short-chain fatty acids (SCFAs), such as butyrate, propionate, and acetate. These metabolites, generated from the fermentation of dietary fiber, have powerful anti-inflammatory and immune-regulating properties. Longevity itself is strongly linked to the abundance of SCFA-producing microbes, including *Clostridium* cluster XIVa, *Ruminococcaceae*, *Akkermansia spp*, and *Christensenellaceae*. With age, however, the gut's microbial diversity begins to decline. The once-stable balance between major phyla shifts: **Firmicutes** decrease while **Bacteroidetes** increase, lowering the Firmicutes-to-Bacteroidetes (F/B) ratio—a critical marker of SCFA production. This age-related dysbiosis does not merely accompany aging; it can actively drive frailty, chronic inflammation, and a decline in resilience.

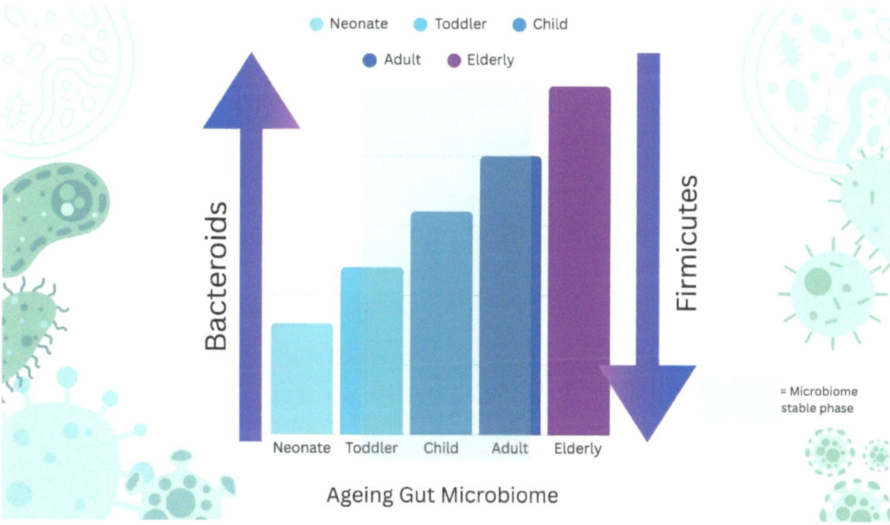

One marker that increases during gut dysbiosis is a cluster of molecules called **SASP factors** (Senescence-Associated Secretory Phenotype). These include cytokines, chemokines, growth factors, proteases, and lipids—tiny messengers that tell your cells how to behave. Some of these messengers are not kind to your skin microbiome. They encourage the rise of **MMPs—matrix metalloproteinases**, enzymes that break down the proteins that keep you youthful: collagen, elastin, fibronectin, and proteoglycans. As these building blocks of the **extracellular matrix** degrade, your skin begins to wrinkle, sag, and lose its elasticity. I feel it, and I try to signal your body, but the imbalance is tricky to fix.

That's why scientists are exploring ways to help me—your microbiome—stay strong and balanced. By nurturing both your gut and your skin microbial communities, it may be possible to slow these premature aging signals. But there's still much to learn about how these distant worlds—the gut, my microbial family, and your skin cells—talk to each other.

For now, I continue my watch, sending tiny signals and trying my best to protect your skin's integrity. With a balanced diet, mindful skincare, and the right microbial allies, we might just age gracefully together.

Gut produces short-chain fatty acids (SCFAs) like butyrate, propionate, and acetate. These molecules:

- Strengthen epithelial tight junctions, reducing "leaky gut"
- Regulate T-regulatory (Treg) cells, maintaining immune tolerance
- Suppress pro-inflammatory cytokines (IL-6, TNF-α, IL-17)
- Promote anti-inflammatory cytokines (IL-10)
- With age, gut microbial diversity often declines:
- Firmicutes decrease, Bacteroidetes increase → lower SCFA production
- Dysbiosis leads to chronic inflammation
- Enzymes like matrix metalloproteinases (MMPs) break down collagen and elastin → wrinkles, sagging, reduced elasticity

Thus, *the story of aging is not written by your genes alone but also by the microbial companions within your gut and on your skin*, **shaping health and longevity from the inside out**.

In short, **what happens in your gut reflects on your skin**.

Aging; increased skin care products and My Challenges

The anti-aging creams and serums you apply daily interact with my home. Many of these products contain preservatives, which keep the product safe from harmful microbes—but they don't distinguish between "good" and "bad." Sometimes, I get disrupted; my balance is altered, and that can affect your skin's health. Certain active ingredients, if not carefully formulated, can also tip the scales, changing the way I function.

But don't worry—I have allies: prebiotics, probiotics, and postbiotics. They help me maintain your skin's natural barrier and resilience. Probiotics like *Lactobacillus* and *Bifidobacterium* are emerging as little warriors, helping slow down the visible signs of aging.

Together, we can:

1. **Keep your skin hydrated:** Combating dryness that often comes with age.
2. **Calm inflammation:** Reducing redness, irritation, and flare-ups.
3. **Smooth texture and reduce fine lines:** Postbiotics help cell turnover rate and collagen production, while probiotics restore balance, making your skin look youthful.
4. **Protect against sun damage:** Helping shield your skin from UV-induced aging.

Remember, my family members change constantly depending on your skin's environment. Genetics, gender, sun exposure, pollution, climate, exercise, stress, sleep, nutrition, and skincare habits—all of these influence me. As you age, microbial imbalances can speed up inflammation, skin fragility, and the signs of aging.

A diverse, balanced microbiome is key to healthy, glowing skin. That's why **microbiome-friendly skincare isn't just a trend—it's an essential part of your anti-aging journey.** Scientists around the world are exploring probiotics and microbiome-targeted treatments as the next frontier in keeping your skin youthful.

So, treat me well, and I'll help you age gracefully—hydrated, balanced, and resilient, one microbial family at a time. By working together, we can slow down **photoaging**, reduce **fine lines**, maintain **skin hydration**, and keep your skin glowing and resilient.

Microbiome-friendly interventions, we can fight back Aging:

- Prebiotics feed the helpful microbes
- Probiotics restore diversity
- Postbiotics reduce oxidative stress and inflammation
- Synbiotics amplify all of the above

Role of Probiotic strains in Anti-ageing process of skin

Lactobacillus brevis (L.brevis) SBC8803

- Improve skin hydration

Nitrosomonas eutropha

- Topical formulations to reduces wrinkles
- *Actinomycetes* - High Facial wrinkling, so have to be replaced with beneficial bacteria

Sphingomonas

- Reduce reactive oxygen species
- Protects solar damage

Lactococcus

- Maintains skin hydration

Nesseria

- Maintains hydration
- Increases skin elasticity

Supporting Healthy Aging

Modern skincare is shifting from simple anti-aging to **microbiome-friendly aging.** Prebiotics, probiotics, and postbiotics can:

- Restore microbial balance
- Support healthy skin barrier
- Reduce oxidative stress
- Protect against premature aging

By caring for me, your skin microbiome, you also care for your skin's resilience and appearance.

Key Takeaways

- Aging alters **skin physiology** (less sebum, altered pH, weaker immunity), reshaping microbial communities.
- Modifying skin physiology during the aging process, such as hydration, sebum secretion, pH, and lipid composition, could help predict changes in microbiota.
- **Early-life colonization** influences immunity and skin health long-term.
- Puberty triggers microbial shifts due to hormones and sebum production.
- Adult microbiome is relatively stable but **site-specific**.
- Older age leads to **reduced diversity**, fragile barriers, and higher disease susceptibility.
- Gut dysbiosis accelerates skin aging through **reduced SCFAs** and chronic inflammation.
- **Prebiotic, probiotic, and postbiotic skincare** helps maintain microbial balance and skin health.

"I grow with you, from your first breath to your final years. Care for me at every stage, and together we can keep your skin strong, radiant, and gracefully aging.

Chapter 3

Skin Gut communication

Me, the messenger

I am your messenger, linking two of your body's largest microbial worlds: your **skin** and your **gut**. Your skin is the first-line barrier to the outer environment, continuously interacting with the vast microbial world. The gastrointestinal (GI) tract is also one of the largest interfaces (30 m^2) between your body and the outer environment. Each hosts trillions of microbial cells, constantly interacting with your immune system. While your skin spans 1.5–2 m^2 and harbours about 10^{12} microbes per cm^2, your gut is even larger—about 30 m^2, containing nearly 10^{14} microbial cells.

Though separate, these two ecosystems communicate continually, shaping **immune responses, inflammation, and overall skin health**.

"My Family Across Two Worlds: Skin and Gut"

I may be small, but I live in a vast, bustling neighbourhood. Your skin is heavily colonized with members of my family—a varied microbial world of bacteria, fungi, and even tiny viruses. But we're not alone here. Your skin is also patrolled by armies of immune cells. Together, we are constantly training these immune soldiers, teaching them when to defend you and when to live peacefully. This training is what keeps your body well.

But my family doesn't only live on the skin. Deep inside you, in your intestinal tract, another vibrant branch of our family thrives. The gut microbiome is even more diverse—home to bacteria, fungi, and protozoa. Many of them are not just harmless passengers but essential workers. They take the complex foods you cannot digest—like tough polysaccharides—and break them down into life-supporting nutrients: **vitamin K, vitamin B12, butyrate, and propionate**.

These metabolites are more than nutrients—they are builders of strength. They help maintain the **epithelial barrier** of the gut, a protective wall that decides what enters your bloodstream and what stays out. When this barrier is intact, your microbiome remains safely in its home, and inflammation is kept under control. But when the barrier is weakened, trouble can spill into the circulation, leading to unwanted inflammation.

So you see, whether on your skin or in your gut, my family works tirelessly—training your immune cells, producing vital nutrients, and keeping barriers strong. We are your hidden allies, quietly shaping your health every day.

Conversations Across the Body – My Distant Relatives

As I mentioned earlier, I don't live in isolation;I am part of a vast network. Recent scientific discoveries reveal something fascinating: my relatives in the gut can influence organs far away, like the **lungs, brain, and even me, the skin**. These conversations are known as the **gut–lung axis, gut–brain axis, and gut–skin axis**. We whisper across distances, shaping your health in ways you may not see.

I am your skin microbiome, but I am never alone. My story is tied to the gut, the lungs, the brain, and the immune cells that weave us together. Caring for your inner world is the surest way to protect me, your outer shield

Your body's defence system—both innate and adaptive immunity—doesn't just watch over you. It also changes my community, deciding who among us thrives or dwindles. Yet this relationship is never one-sided. We, your microbes, can also guide your immune system, training it to respond with balance or, sometimes, with too much force.

When your **gut falls into dysbiosis**, I feel it here on your surface. The balance of my community breaks, and skin homeostasis is lost. This disruption shows up as inflammatory skin conditions you know well: **psoriasis, atopic dermatitis, rosacea, seborrheic dermatitis, dandruff, alopecia areata, hidradenitis suppurativa.** My harmony fades, and your skin suffers.

Food plays a bigger role in this than you might imagine. Certain ingredients in your diet can weaken the **intestinal barrier**, opening small gateways. Through these cracks, members of my gut relatives can slip into the bloodstream. When this happens, the immune system reacts, and I feel the ripple effects on your skin.

Lifestyle choices—your food, hygiene, and even stress—combined with your unique genetics, all shape how tolerant your immune system is toward me and my fellow commensal microbes. A balanced life helps your immune system see us as allies, not invaders. But when that balance tips, inflammation rises, and diseases emerge.

The connection between the your skin and gut seems to be mediated by the host immune system.

When the Walls Weaken

I am your skin microbiome, and I must tell you about a danger I often sense coming from far away—your gut. You see, your gut's epithelial barrier is like a fortress wall. It decides what can pass through and what must stay out. When it is strong, I live in peace. But when this wall weakens, cracks begin to appear.

Through these cracks, parts of your gut microbiota—tiny fragments, toxins, and metabolites—slip into the bloodstream. To your immune system, these look like invaders. Immediately, alarms go on, and your body's soldiers rush into action. What begins as protection quickly turns into a storm: **inflammation.**

And here's the truth—what happens in the gut does not stay in the gut. The inflammation spills outward, reaching me here on the skin. It disrupts my community, tipping the balance between my friendly members and the opportunistic troublemakers. The harmony we once shared breaks down.

In this chaos, the inflammatory messengers from your gut combine with local changes in my world. Together, they accelerate processes like **matrix metalloproteinase (MMP) activation**, breaking down your skin's supportive framework—collagen, elastin, fibronectin. Slowly, you notice it: fine lines, wrinkles, sagging, irritation. The face you see in the mirror reflects not only the years but also the turmoil within.

But here is the hope: when you strengthen the gut barrier, you strengthen me. A diet rich in fiber, polyphenols, and prebiotics nourishes your gut microbes. Probiotics introduce new allies. Reduced stress and good sleep calm the immune storms. When your gut wall stands tall again, inflammation settles, and I too regain balance.

The walls between gut and skin are invisible, but we are deeply connected. Care for one home, and you protect the other. Together, we can age with resilience, not fragility.

Two Worlds, One Connection (Gut-Skin Axis)

Your gut microbes ferment fibre into **short-chain fatty acids (SCFAs)** like acetate, propionate, and butyrate. These molecules:

- Strengthen intestinal tight junctions, reducing "leaky gut"
- Modulate **T-regulatory (Treg) cells** to maintain immune tolerance
- Reduce pro-inflammatory cytokines (IL-6, TNF-α, IL-17)
- Increase anti-inflammatory cytokines (IL-10)

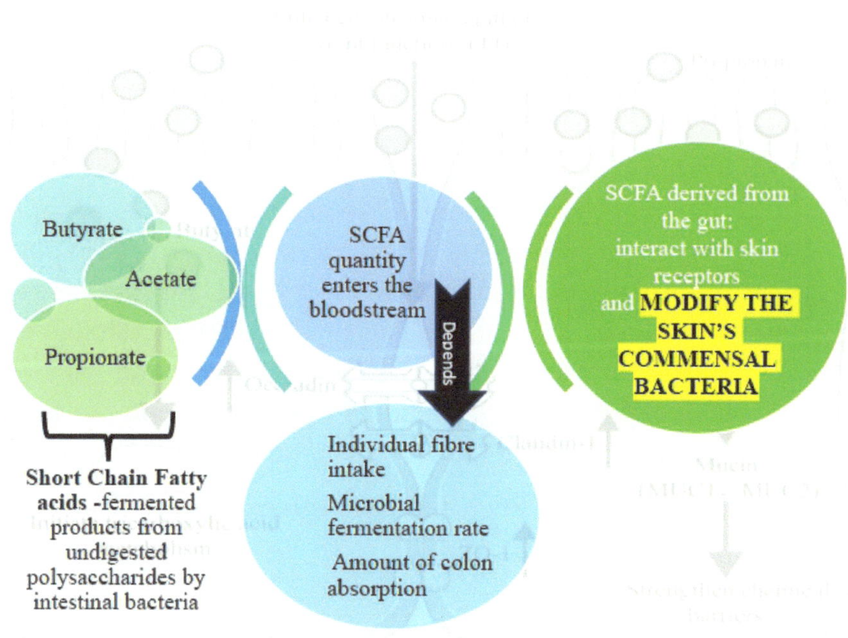

By doing so, SCFAs indirectly influence your **skin immune responses**, reducing risks of conditions like **psoriasis, atopic dermatitis, and acne**.

When Gut Dysbiosis Hits

A disturbed gut microbiome (dysbiosis) can trigger skin problems:

- **Leaky gut:** bacterial fragments like lipopolysaccharides (LPS) enter circulation, promoting systemic inflammation
- **Altered metabolites:** loss of SCFA producers and overgrowth of pathobionts disrupt immune balance
- **Inflammatory cascades:** Th17 and Th1 responses intensify, directly affecting skin

Clinical observations reveal:

- **Psoriasis:** reduced *Akkermansia muciniphila* and *Faecalibacterium prausnitzii* correlate with inflammation
- **Atopic dermatitis:** lower gut microbial diversity in early life, especially *Bifidobacterium spp.*

- **Rosacea:** linked to SIBO (small intestinal bacterial overgrowth), producing pro-inflammatory metabolites.

Beyond Food: The Hygiene Hypothesis

Modern life has reduced exposure to environmental microbes. The more urbanized and clean you tend to keep your body, the better it is for me to harbor you. The hygiene hypothesis stating reduced exposure to microbes through modern health practices leads to increased inflammatory diseases in the urbanized society. People living in non-urbanized environments (indigenous people and farming environments), exposed to a vast variety of environmental microbial flora, are usually not characterized by inflammatory diseases.

Over-sanitization may **weaken immune tolerance**, predisposing to atopic diseases and asthma:

- Children raised on farms often show lower rates of asthma and eczema
- Controlled microbial exposure strengthens immune regulation and balances skin responses.

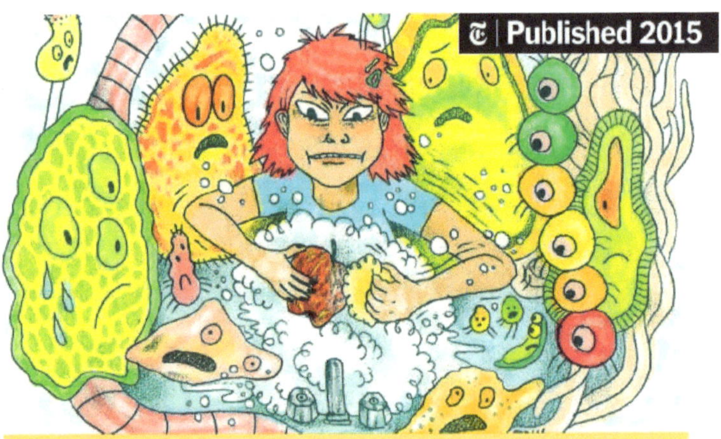

Invite Some Germs to Dinner - The New York Times, 2015

Bidirectional Communication: Skin ↔ Gut

Communication isn't one-way: The gut–skin axis of your body exists bidirectionally and is not only governed by diet and your lifestyle.

- **UVB exposure** increases vitamin D → enhances gut microbial diversity (relative abundance of good bacteria as *Lachnospira spp* and *Fusicatenibacter* genera) and SCFA production.
- **Atopic dermatitis** weakens the skin barrier → allows allergens (like peanuts) to sensitize the gut immune system (immunoglobulin E (IgE)-mediated cell expansion in the gut) → food allergies

This constant dialogue means **gut and skin co-regulate immunity and inflammation**.

The Food You Eat, The Skin I Wear

I've been whispering secrets about your gut, your immune system, and me. Now, let me share one of the biggest truths: the food you eat writes directly on the canvas of your skin.

Let's start with the **Western diet**. When your meals are heavy in fats and processed foods, your gut family tips out of balance. The harmony between *Firmicutes* and *Bacteroidetes* shifts, leading to **intestinal dysbiosis**. And when the gut falters, I feel it. My balance breaks, and your skin begins to show signs of stress.

This same Western diet doesn't just affect me; it fuels the rise of **immune-mediated diseases (IMIDs)**—conditions like rheumatoid arthritis, psoriasis, and atopic dermatitis. When your immune system becomes overactive, I am caught in the crossfire, showing redness, irritation, or flare-ups.

Some foods carry hidden secrets. Take the **nightshade family**—tomatoes, potatoes, eggplants, and peppers. They hold small amounts of alkaloids like glycoalkaloids, alpha-tomatine, and capsaicin. In excess, these can weaken your gut barrier, opening cracks that allow troublemakers to spill into circulation. I notice this immediately—your skin becomes vulnerable, inflamed, less radiant.

Then, there's **gluten**. For some, it is harmless. But for others, gluten cracks open the gates of the gut and brings storms to the skin. In **celiac**

disease and gluten sensitivity, immune confusion arises. The skin suffers—sometimes as **dermatitis herpetiformis**, an itchy rash that only quiets when gluten disappears from the diet. For some it takes months; for others, years. And beyond celiac disease, other autoimmune conditions, like psoriasis, also feel the weight of gluten intolerance.

Thus, what you eat profoundly shapes my world:

- **High-fibre diets** → boost SCFA production, protecting gut and skin
- **Western diets** (high-fat, high-sugar) → increase Firmicutes, reduce Bacteroidetes → inflammation
- **Gluten** → can loosen intestinal junctions in sensitive individuals, worsening autoimmune-related skin diseases
- **Nightshades** (tomatoes, potatoes, eggplants, peppers) → may increase gut permeability and trigger inflammation
- **Polyphenols** (green tea, berries, cocoa) → feed beneficial microbes and enhance SCFA production

So, you see, every bite you take reaches me, even if it starts in the gut. Your food can nourish the walls that protect us or weaken them. Your diet can calm inflammation or stir it into a storm. Remember, I wear your choices—I am the skin you see in the mirror.

Diet as a Modulator of the Gut–Skin Axis:

The amount of fibre intake, microbial fermentation rate, the amount of SCFA absorption by the colon determines the quantity of SCFA entering your bloodstream. All these compounds, which are derived from the gut, interact with skin receptors and could directly affect the skin or modify the skin's commensal bacteria. The gut-skin axis underscores the profound connection between internal health and external appearance.

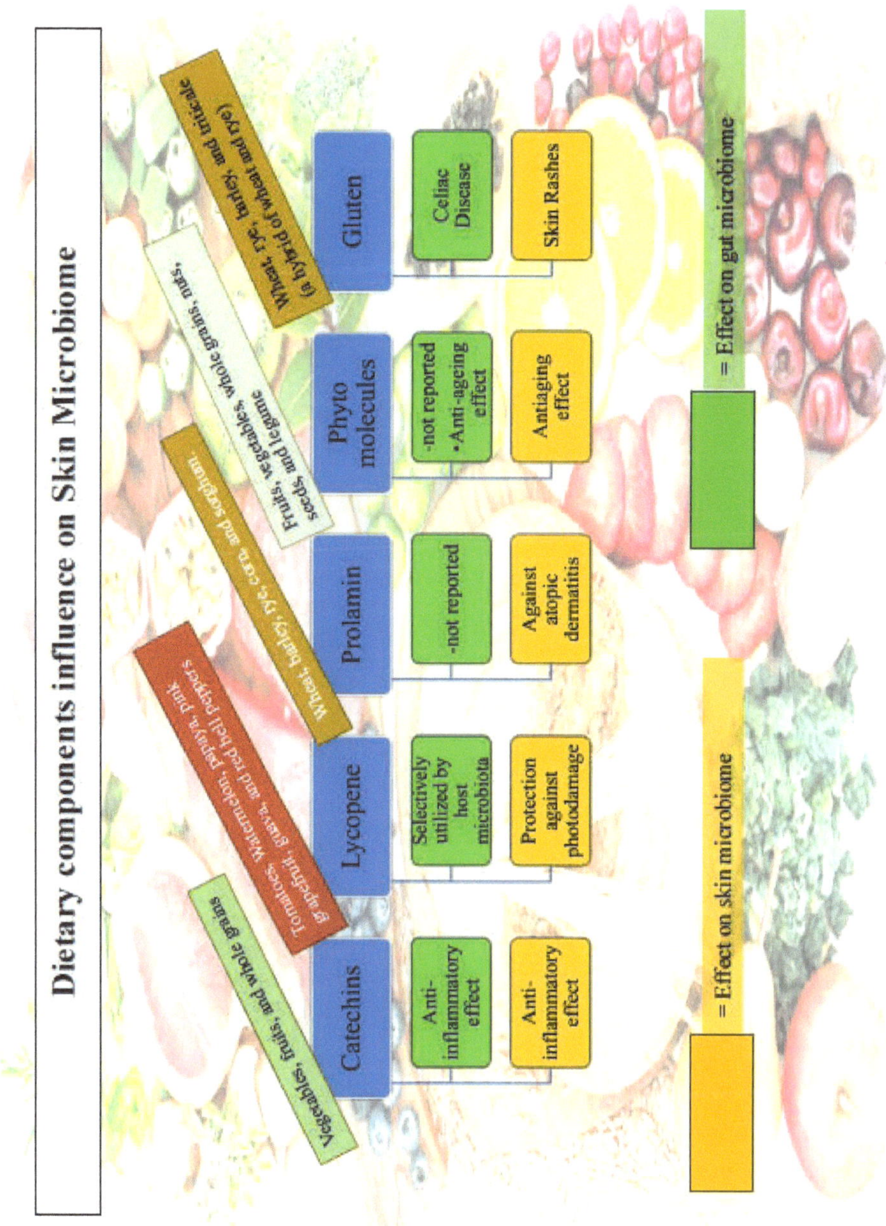
Dietary components influence on Skin Microbiome
Vegetables, fruits, and whole grains
Tomatoes, Watermelon, papaya, pink grapefruit, guava, and red bell peppers
Wheat, barley, rye, corn, and sorghum
Fruits, vegetables, whole grains, nuts, seeds and legume
Wheat, rye, barley, and triticale (a hybrid of wheat and rye)
Catechins
Lycopene
Prolamin
Phyto molecules
Gluten
Anti-inflammatory effect
Selectively utilized by host microbiota
-not reported
-not reported •Anti-ageing effect
Celiac Disease
Anti-inflammatory effect
Protection against photodamage
Against atopic dermatitis
Antiaging effect
Skin Rashes
= Effect on skin microbiome
= Effect on gut microbiome

Supporting the Gut–Skin Axis

Strategies to maintain balance: Maintaining a healthy gut through a balanced diet and lifestyle can have significant benefits for your skin's health and appearance.

1. **Eating a balanced diet:** Anti-inflammatory diet → fibre, omega-3s, antioxidants. Limiting processed foods, sugars, and unhealthy fats.
2. **Consuming 3P's: Probiotics, Prebiotics, Postbiotics**, along with prebiotics (fibres that nourish beneficial bacteria), can help rebalance the gut microbiome and support both gut and skin health. Postbiotics (bioactive compounds made by probiotic bacteria when they ferment fibre).
    - **Probiotics:** Beneficial bacteria in fermented foods or supplements like *Lactobacillus rhamnosus GG* reduce atopic dermatitis in children
    - **Prebiotics:** Fibres that nourish beneficial bacteria. Like inulin, fructo-oligosaccharides feed beneficial microbes.
    - **Postbiotics:** Bioactive compounds made by probiotic bacteria when they ferment fibre. Like butyrate and propionate supplements reduce skin inflammation
3. **Stress management** → cortisol disrupts gut and skin barriers
4. **Hydration** → supports mucosal surfaces and skin elasticity

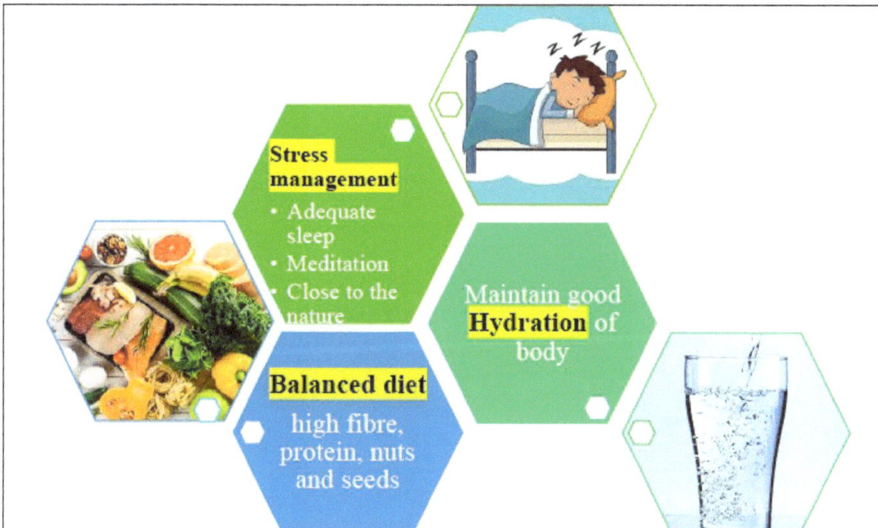
Stress management
• Adequate sleep
• Meditation
• Close to the nature
Maintain good Hydration of body
Balanced diet
high fibre, protein, nuts and seeds

Key factors for maintaining the Gut-Skin Axis

Key Takeaways

The **gut–skin axis** relies on microbial metabolites, immune signalling, and systemic inflammation.

- Gut dysbiosis drives skin conditions via leaky gut, LPS release, and altered T-cell responses.
- Diet, lifestyle, and environment strongly shape microbial balance.
- Skin health can influence gut health through vitamin D and allergen exposure.
- Probiotics, prebiotics, and postbiotics offer therapeutic potential in skin disorders.
- Holistic care—balanced diet, microbial exposure, hydration, stress control—supports both gut and skin health.

"I am your living link, carrying biochemical whispers between gut and skin. When harmony thrives within me, your skin reflects it with strength and clarity. Care for me from the inside, and I will keep your outside glowing."

Chapter 4
Skin Nerve communication

Me, the messenger

When Nerves Whisper Through My World

The studies support the idea that your gut and skin interact with one another via diet, the metabolites produced due to resident microbial flora as well as through the neuroendocrine pathways, and the central nervous system.

Did you know that I don't just live with immune cells and barrier proteins? I also live shoulder to shoulder with a vast web of **nerves**. They weave through your skin like roots beneath the soil, carrying signals between me and your brain. This is what scientists call the **skin neuro–immune pathway**.

When you feel a gentle touch, a sharp prick, or even an itch, it's because these nerves have listened to me and my environment. We microbes can activate them, sending tiny electrical whispers that travel all the way to your brain.

But the conversation doesn't end there. Your brain speaks back. Stress, anxiety, or even joy can send molecules—like **cortisol, neuropeptides, and neurotransmitters**—down through your nerves, changing the way I behave. Sometimes stress makes me restless, tipping the balance toward inflammation. That's why breakouts or rashes often appear during stressful times.

Certain molecules—**substance P, CGRP, acetylcholine**—are messengers that connect your nerves with immune cells and me. They can either calm the system or stir it into irritation, itching, and redness. This is why conditions like **atopic dermatitis, psoriasis, and chronic itch** are not just skin problems; they are neuro-immune conversations gone astray.

Likewise, in 2011, Bowe and Logan described the **gut–brain–skin axis**, highlighting how stress, diet, and gut microbes together influence acne severity.

So, every time your skin tingles, itches, or flares, remember—it's not just me. It's a dialogue between your **nerves, immune system, brain, and microbes**. The neuro-cutaneous pathway is my hotline to your mind.

Care for your stress, nourish your body, and I will reflect it. Because the calmer your brain, the calmer I am on your skin.

The Food That Speaks to My Nerves

I am your skin microbiome, and today I'll tell you about how every meal you take doesn't just feed your gut—it also whispers to my nerves.

When you eat a fiber-rich diet, your gut relatives break it down into **short-chain fatty acids**. These molecules travel like peacekeepers, calming inflammation and strengthening barriers. With strong walls, fewer irritants reach me, and my nerves stay calm.

But when your plate is full of processed foods, sugar, or unhealthy fats, your gut barrier weakens. Small fragments—like bacterial lipopolysaccharides—slip into your blood. When they arrive in my world, they poke at immune cells and nerve endings, sparking a fire: redness, itch, sometimes even pain. This is **neurogenic inflammation**—a flare born not from outside but from food choices within.

Some foods even hold direct keys to the nervous system. **Nightshades** (tomatoes, potatoes, peppers, eggplants) carry alkaloids that may irritate barriers and awaken nerves. **Gluten**, for some, acts as a trigger, sending itchy signals through my pathways.

Diet → Gut Microbiome → Skin Neuro–Pathway

1. **Leaky Gut & Neuroinflammation**
   - Gut barrier breakdown allows bacterial products (like LPS) into circulation.
   - These molecules can sensitize peripheral nerves and immune cells in the skin.
2. **Neuroactive Metabolites**
   - Some gut bacteria ferment foods into **neuroactive compounds** (e.g., serotonin precursors, GABA, dopamine-related molecules).
   - These can affect both central nervous system (brain) and **cutaneous nerves** (skin).
3. **Dietary Triggers of Neurogenic Inflammation in Skin**
   - Gluten, glycoalkaloids (tomatoes, potatoes, peppers), and high sugar → increase permeability, activate immune & neural pathways → worsen itch, burning, flare-ups.
   - Omega-3 fatty acids, polyphenols, probiotics → calm neuroinflammation, reduce nerve hyper-reactivity.
4. **Result**
   - Diet influences **neuro-immune-microbiome crosstalk** → alters skin sensations (itch, pain, tingling) and inflammatory conditions (psoriasis, atopic dermatitis, rosacea).

And yet, there is balance. **Omega-3s, antioxidants, and polyphenols** from fruits, fish, and plants soothe me. They quiet the nerve activity, reduce stress signals, and restore harmony. Even the gut microbes transform foods into **neuroactive chemicals**—like serotonin and GABA—that keep both your brain and my nerves balanced.

So, when you choose your food, you're not just feeding your body. You're shaping a conversation between your gut, your nerves, and me—your skin. Every bite is a message, and I translate it into the way you look and feel.

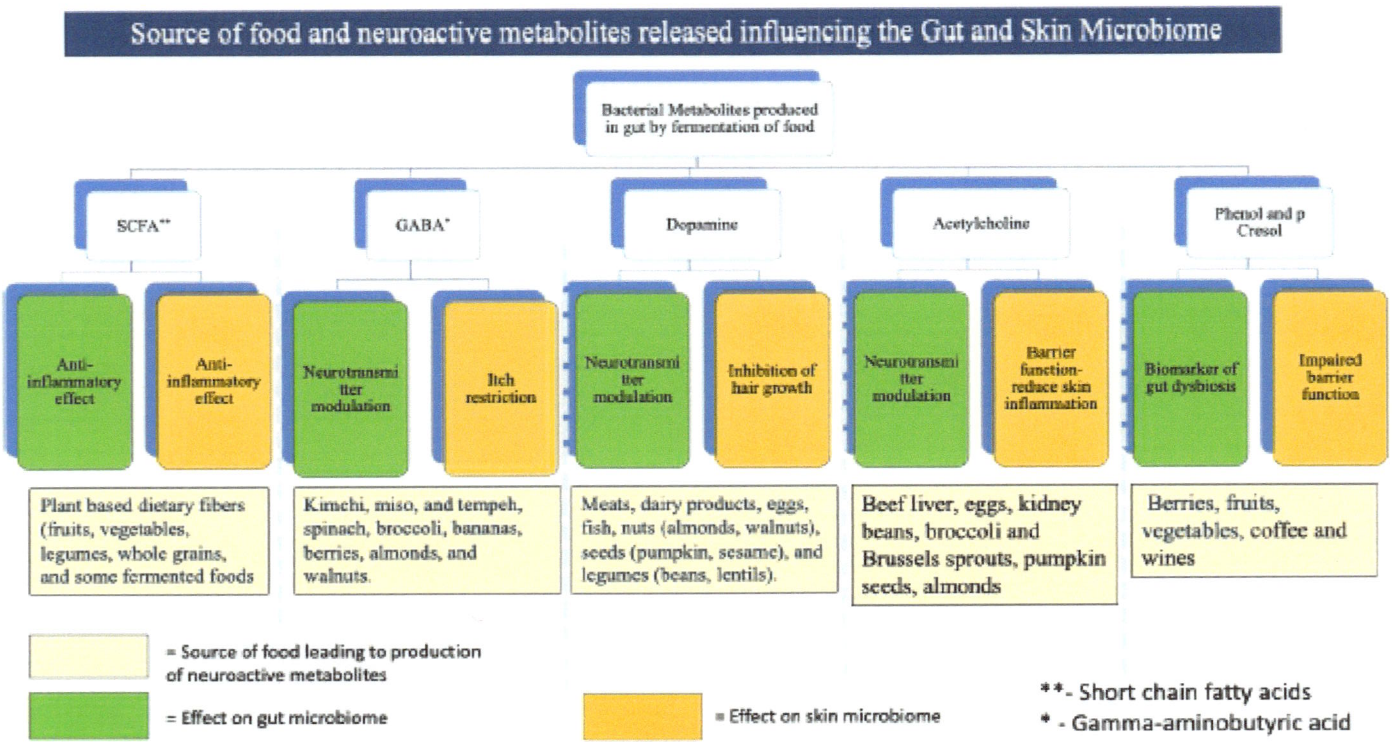
Source of food and neuroactive metabolites released influencing the Gut and Skin Microbiome
Bacterial Metabolites produced in gut by fermentation of food
SCFA**
GABA*
Dopamine
Acetylcholine
Phenol and p Cresol
Anti-inflammatory effect
Anti-inflammatory effect
Neurotransmitter modulation
Itch restriction
Neurotransmitter modulation
Inhibition of hair growth
Neurotransmitter modulation
Barrier function- reduce skin inflammation
Biomarker of gut dysbiosis
Impaired barrier function
Plant based dietary fibers (fruits, vegetables, legumes, whole grains, and some fermented foods
Kimchi, miso, and tempeh, spinach, broccoli, bananas, berries, almonds, and walnuts.
Meats, dairy products, eggs, fish, nuts (almonds, walnuts), seeds (pumpkin, sesame), and legumes (beans, lentils).
Beef liver, eggs, kidney beans, broccoli and Brussels sprouts, pumpkin seeds, almonds
Berries, fruits, vegetables, coffee and wines
= Source of food leading to production of neuroactive metabolites
= Effect on gut microbiome
= Effect on skin microbiome
**- Short chain fatty acids
* - Gamma-aminobutyric acid

Key Messages – When Food Whispers Through My Nerves

1. **Skin and brain are linked** through the **skin neuro–pathway**; nerves carry signals both ways between microbes and the brain.
2. **Microbes produce neuroactive compounds that can affect both the central nervous system (brain) and cutaneous nerves (skin).**
3. **Stress and emotions** (via cortisol, neuropeptides, neurotransmitters) directly influence skin behavior, often triggering flare-ups.
4. **Fiber-rich foods** → gut microbes produce short-chain fatty acids (SCFAs) that strengthen barriers and calm inflammation.
5. **Processed foods, sugar, and unhealthy fats** → weaken the gut barrier, allow bacterial fragments (LPS) to irritate nerves and immune cells → flare-ups.
6. **Trigger foods**: Nightshades (tomatoes, potatoes, peppers, eggplants) and gluten can worsen neurogenic inflammation in some people.
7. **Healing foods**: Omega-3s, antioxidants, polyphenols, and probiotics reduce nerve sensitivity, calm the skin, and restore balance.
8. **Every bite is a message**—diet shapes the gut–nerve–skin conversation, influencing whether your skin glows or flares.

**"Every meal, every thought, every feeling shapes me.
Care for your gut, calm your mind, and I will keep your skin healthy and radiant."**

Chapter 5

Acne

My popping buddy

Acne – My Troubled Neighbourhood

The **skin microbiome**, living mostly in your oily zones, is unique in itself. Sometimes, life gets chaotic in my neighbourhoods—especially when acne develops. Acne, commonly termed as 'pimples', is a chronic inflammatory skin disease involving the pilosebaceous units of your skin.

How Acne Starts

Acne is a **chronic inflammatory disease** (disharmony of my home) of the pilosebaceous unit.

Causes include:

- Microbial dysbiosis: imbalance between *Cutibacterium acnes* and other microbes
- Immune overreaction
- Excess sebum production
- Hormonal influences

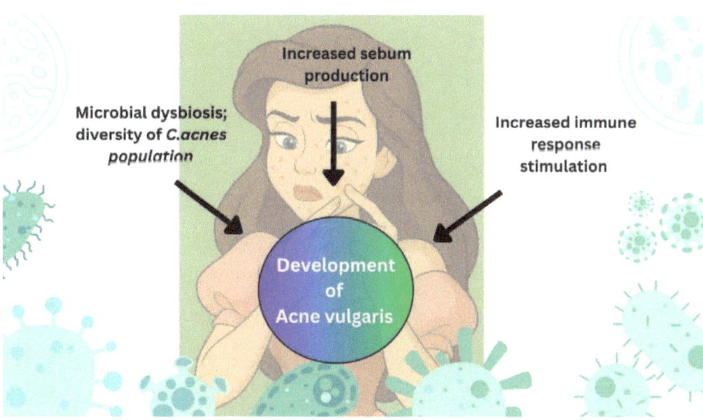

Microbial Cast - When Oil Meets Microbes

Among my family, *Cutibacterium acnes* is the key microbe associated with acne vulgaris. It is not just its presence but its **overgrowth, virulence factors, and strain variability** that drive inflammation and acne lesions.

Sebaceous (oily) sites such as the face, back, and chest are rich in free fatty acids because sebaceous glands secrete large amounts of sebum. This makes these regions acidic and nutrient-dense, providing an ideal niche for microbes like *Cutibacterium spp.* that metabolize sebum.

Inside the **anaerobic pilosebaceous units**, *C. acnes* produces lipases that hydrolyze triglycerides in sebum into **free fatty acids (FFAs)**, including **propionic acid**. These metabolites lower pH further, disrupt the epidermal barrier, and serve as **pro-inflammatory mediators**. FFAs can activate **Toll-like receptors (TLR2)** on keratinocytes and immune cells, triggering cytokine release (e.g., IL-1β, IL-8, TNF-α), which drives the recruitment of neutrophils and initiation of local inflammation.

Certain *C. acnes* strains carry **virulence genes** encoding Christie-Atkins-Munch-Petersen (CAMP) factors, porphyrins, and enzymes that contribute to **oxidative stress** and **biofilm formation**. These factors promote follicular plugging, comedone formation, and a chronic inflammatory environment.

While *C. acnes* dominates, ***Staphylococcus species*** also influence the balance. *Staphylococcus epidermidis*, although generally a commensal, can become opportunistic; it competes with *C. acnes* by producing antimicrobial peptides (AMPs) but also contributes lipases that liberate free fatty acids (FFAs). *Staphylococcus aureus*, on the other hand, is strongly associated with exacerbations, producing toxins and superantigens that worsen inflammation.

The interaction between **host sebum composition, microbial metabolism, and the immune response** determines whether skin remains clear or develops acne. Increased androgen levels stimulate sebaceous gland activity, producing more triglyceride-rich sebum, which in turn fuels microbial overgrowth.

Thus, acne is not merely a cosmetic problem—it is a **multifactorial disease involving the sebaceous gland, *Cutibacterium* strains, skin immune system, and neuroendocrine signals**.

- ***C. acnes***: thrives on oil, can trigger inflammation.
- ***S. epidermidis***: usually protective, may decrease in dysbiosis
- ***Malassezia***: minor contributor in oily skin

→ Skin microbial dysbiosis commonly observed in patients with acne

From Blackheads to Scars: The Acne Story I Witness Every Day

I usually protect your skin and keep things in balance. But sometimes, changes in oil (sebum), hormones, and blocked pores invite troublemakers into our community.

a. **The First Visitors — Primary Lesions (Non-inflammatory)**
   Meet the Comedone cousins!

   - **Open comedones (Blackheads):** These like to sit in wide pores. Their contents get exposed to air, turning dark because of oxidized keratin and lipids.
   - **Closed comedones (Whiteheads):** These are the shy ones, staying beneath the skin's surface, forming small white or skin-colored bumps.

   "I can usually manage these two — they're annoying, but not too dangerous."

b. **The Unruly Guests — Inflammatory Lesions**

- **Papules:** "Here come the red, raised, angry bumps. They bring tenderness and start causing discomfort."
- **Pustules:** "Papules often invite pus to the party — now they have yellow/white heads, making them hard to ignore."

"I start to struggle as these fiery guests disturb the peace."

c. **The Troublemakers — Severe/Deep Lesions**

- **Nodules:** "Big, firm, and painful, these invaders dig deep into the dermis, leaving long-lasting marks."
- **Cysts:** "Worse still, cysts arrive — swollen, pus-filled, sometimes merging together, threatening abscess formation."

"At this stage, the community is in chaos, and I can't restore order alone — doctors must step in."

d. **The Aftermath — Sequelae**

- **Scarring:** "The worst scars left behind — tiny pits like *ice-picks*, rolling waves, or thick keloids."
- **Post-inflammatory hyperpigmentation (PIH):** "In darker skin, these guests leave brownish patches even after the pimples are gone."

I usually keep peace and balance, but sometimes, things get out of control in our neighbourhood called the **pilosebaceous unit**. That's when acne shows up!

Let me introduce you to three characters who live here: Mild, Moderate, and Severe."

a. **Mild Acne** "When balance tips just a little, you see comedones — blackheads and whiteheads. They're my playful cousins who like to clog pores. Sometimes, they bring a couple of tiny pimples, but they usually don't cause much trouble. I can still manage the peace at this stage."

b. **Moderate Acne** "But then, things heat up. More of my cousins (papules and pustules) arrive, red and inflamed. A few **nodules** sneak in too, making it harder for me to maintain harmony. You begin to notice your skin feels tender, and I start struggling to keep balance."

c. **Severe Acne** "And finally comes the storm. **Nodules and cysts** take over the neighbourhood, digging deep into the skin. They leave behind scars and dark stains as their footprints. At this point, I can't fix the chaos alone — we need medical help to restore balance."

"What You Eat Reflects on Me" — The Gut–Skin Story by Your Skin Microbiome

I, your **skin microbiome,** live on the surface of your skin, protecting you from harmful invaders and keeping your barrier strong. But my health is not just about what happens on the outside — it is deeply tied to my cousin, the **gut microbiome**.

Decades ago, in the **1960s**, doctors tried using *Lactobacillus species* in acne patients and noticed improvements. Back then, it was just a hunch. But now, science confirms what I always knew: *your diet and gut health directly influence me — and your acne.*

Diet Shapes the Gut Microbiota

When you eat a diet rich in **fiber, fruits, and vegetables**, your gut microbiota becomes more diverse. Beneficial bacteria like ***Lactobacilli*** and ***Bifidobacteria*** flourish, producing short-chain fatty acids (SCFAs) such as butyrate, propionate, and acetate. These molecules calm inflammation and strengthen your intestinal barrier.

But when your diet is high in **refined sugars, dairy, and processed foods**, balance is lost. The gut barrier weakens, allowing microbial products (like **lipopolysaccharides, LPS**) to leak into circulation. These pro-inflammatory signals reach me, disturb my balance, and trigger acne flares.

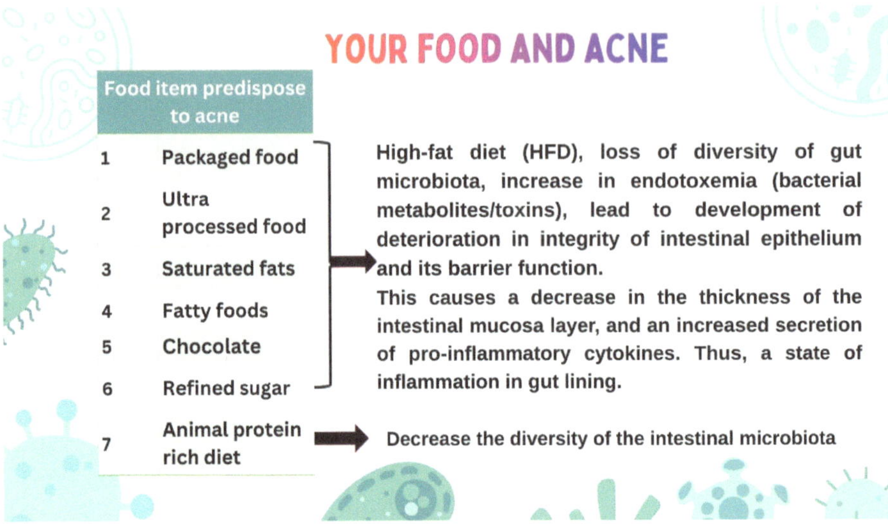

Evidence from Research

Studies show that people with **acne vulgaris** have a **distinct gut microbial profile**:

- **Decreased microbial diversity**
- **Reduced Firmicutes**
- **Increased Bacteroides** (linked with inflammation)
- **Lower levels of *Lactobacilli* and *Bifidobacteria*** (important for gut–skin harmony)

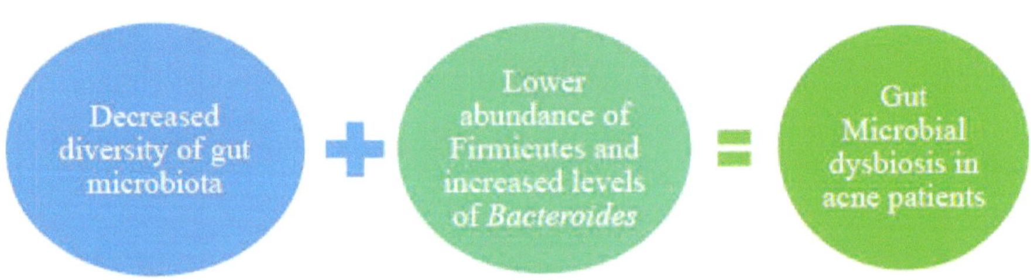

More recent clinical studies confirm that restoring gut health through diet or probiotics can improve acne outcomes. Scientists are now exploring **oral and topical probiotics** to restore harmony. Imagine —

beneficial microbes applied directly to me, or swallowed to help my gut cousin — both working together to fight acne naturally.

"What you eat reflects on your skin." By feeding your gut microbiome well, you support me, your skin microbiome — and together we can keep acne at bay.

Treatment and Microbiome Support in Acne Vulgaris

When acne gets out of control, doctors step in with treatments. But not all treatments are kind to me, your skin microbiome. Let me walk you through how therapies work — and how we can keep our microbial family balanced."

A. **Topical Treatments (First line for mild–moderate acne)**

- **Benzoyl peroxide** → kills *Cutibacterium acnes* (the acne-associated bacteria) and reduces inflammation.
- **Salicylic acid** → unclogs pores by dissolving keratin plugs.
- **Topical retinoids (adapalene, tretinoin)** → normalize follicular turnover, prevent comedones.
- **Topical antibiotics (clindamycin, erythromycin)** → used in more inflamed cases, but should be combined with benzoyl peroxide to prevent resistance.

B. **Systemic Treatments (for moderate–severe or resistant acne)**

- **Oral antibiotics (doxycycline, minocycline, tetracycline)** → reduce *C. acnes* and inflammation, but must be used short-term to avoid resistance and gut dysbiosis.
- **Hormonal therapies (oral contraceptives, spironolactone)** → regulate sebum production in females with hormonally driven acne.
- **Isotretinoin** → the "last-resort" vitamin A derivative that shrinks sebaceous glands, normalizes keratinization, and reduces *C. acnes* drastically. Highly effective but can strongly disrupt me (the microbiome) and has notable side effects.

C. **Microbiome-Friendly Approaches** (emerging supportive care)

- **Prebiotic or probiotic creams** → nurture beneficial skin microbes, restore balance after harsh treatments.
- **Nutricosmetics** → supplements containing *Lactobacillus* or *Bifidobacterium* to support gut–skin harmony.

D. **Dietary of Insights**

- **Gut imbalance affects me:** Fewer *Lactobacilli* & *Bifidobacteria*, more Bacteroides = more acne.
- **Dietary support** → high in **fiber, omega-3 fatty acids, and antioxidants**, promoting gut health and lowering systemic inflammation.
- **Probiotics help:** *Lactobacillus rhamnosus* GG can calm my chaos.
- **Diet matters:** Skim milk and high-glycemic foods stir unrest; fiber, anti-inflammatory foods, and omega-3s soothe me.

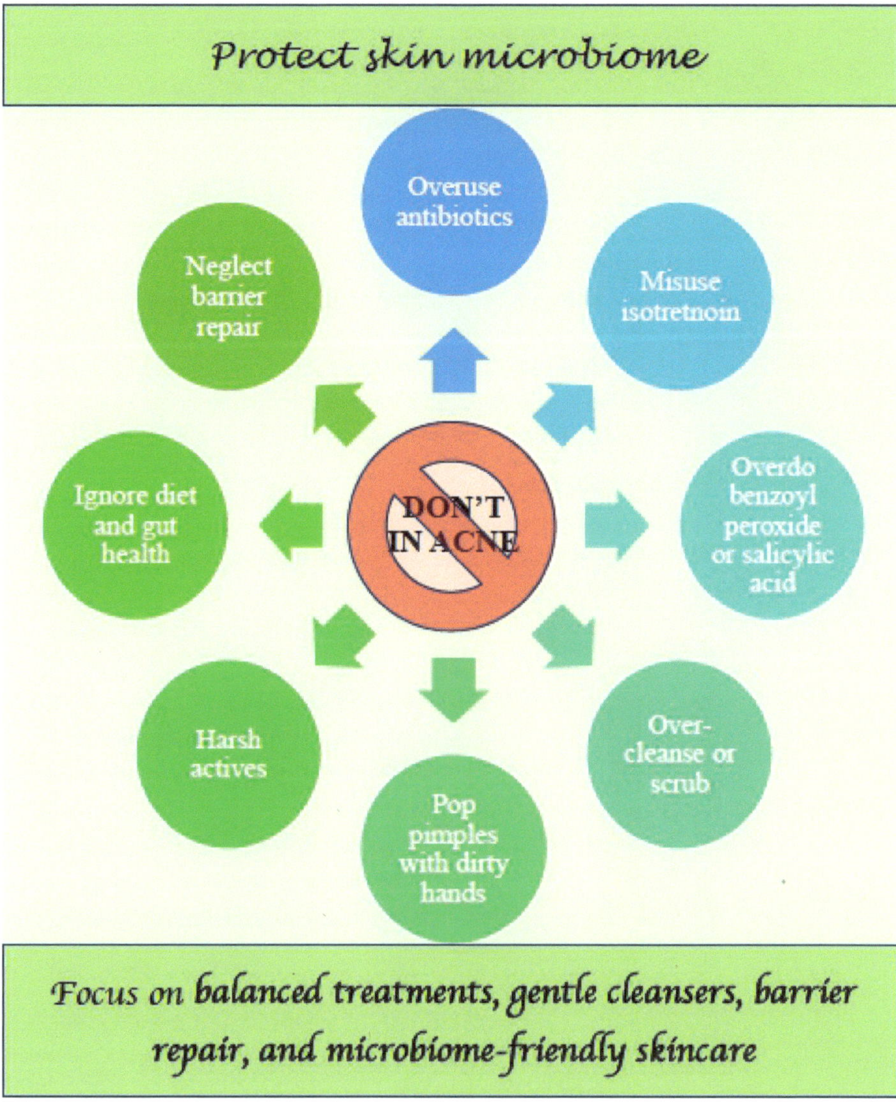
Protect skin microbiome
Overuse antibiotics
Misuse isotretnoin
Overdo benzoyl peroxide or salicylic acid
Over-cleanse or scrub
Pop pimples with dirty hands
Harsh actives
Ignore diet and gut health
Neglect barrier repair
DON'T IN ACNE
Focus on balanced treatments, gentle cleansers, barrier repair, and microbiome-friendly skincare

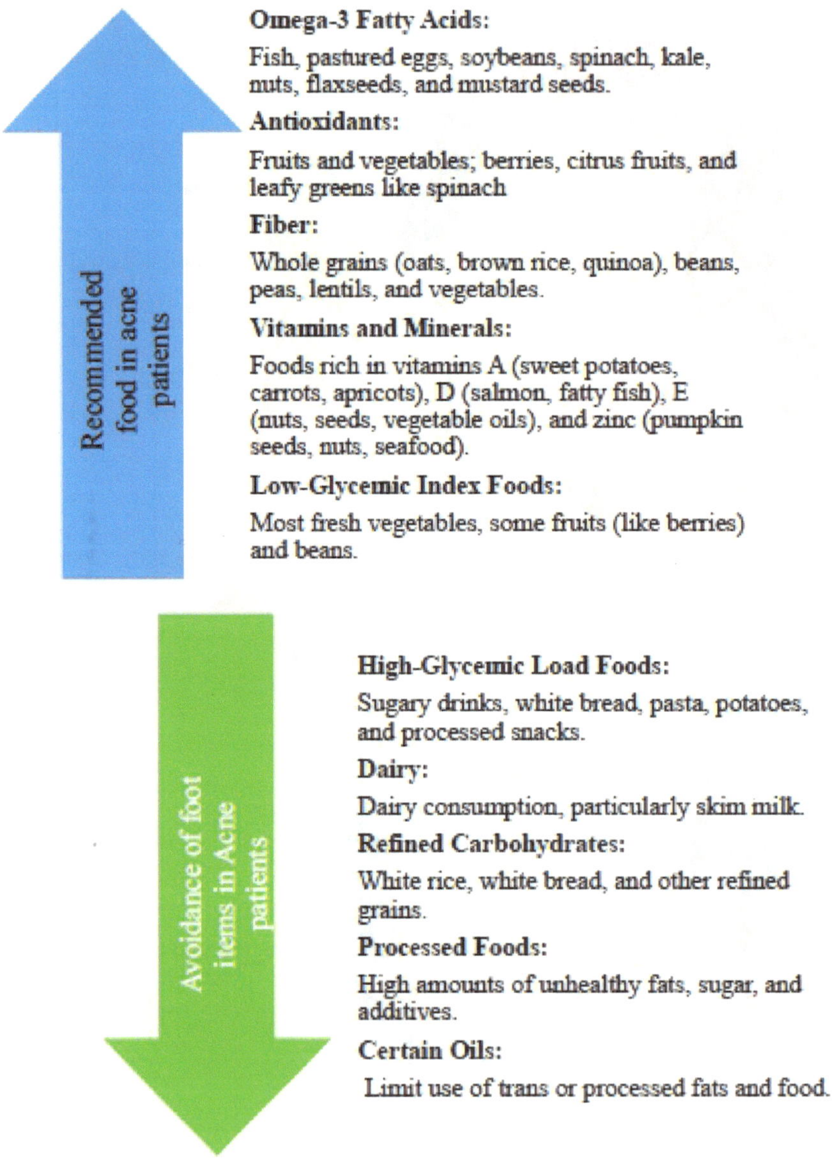

Key Message

1. **Acne** is chronic inflammation of the **pilosebaceous unit**.
2. **Main causes:** microbial imbalance, excess sebum, hormones, immune overreaction.

3. **Key microbes:**
   - *Cutibacterium acnes* – major trigger of inflammation.
   - *Staphylococcus epidermidis* – usually protective, sometimes opportunistic.
   - *Staphylococcus aureus* – worsens flare-ups.
4. **Lesion stages:**
   - Mild – blackheads, whiteheads.
   - Moderate – papules, pustules.
   - Severe – nodules, cysts, scars.
5. **Gut–skin link:** unhealthy diet → gut dysbiosis → acne flares.
6. **Better foods:** fiber, fruits, veggies, omega-3s, probiotics.
7. **Avoid:** sugar, dairy, high-glycemic foods.
8. **Treatments:**
   - Topical – benzoyl peroxide, salicylic acid, retinoids, mild antibiotics.
   - Systemic – oral antibiotics, hormones, isotretinoin.
9. **Microbiome care:** use probiotic creams, gentle cleansers, and gut-friendly diets.
10. **Core message:** keep **skin + gut microbes in balance** to prevent and calm acne.

Acne is really a signal from your microbial world.

"I am the tiny voice beneath your skin. When my world loses balance, pimples appear as my signal. Nourish me, care for my gut cousins, and together, we can keep your skin calm and clear."

Chapter 6

Atopic Dermatitis

The Itchy Tale of a Broken Barrier

I, your skin microbiome, have lived with you since birth, protecting, training, and guiding your immune system. But when the balance in my world is disrupted, I sometimes become part of a story filled with itch, redness, and discomfort — the story of **Atopic Dermatitis (AD)**.

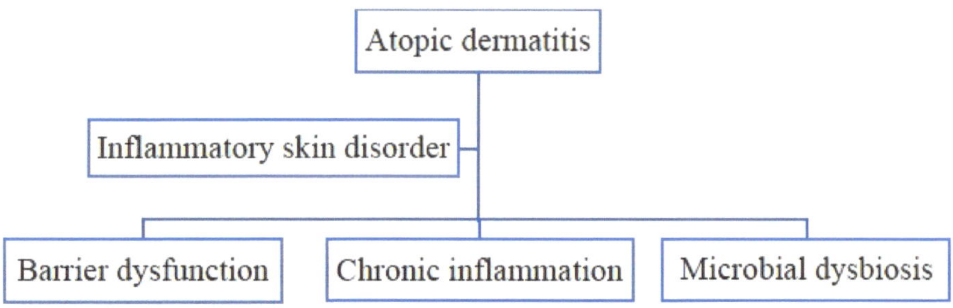

Atopic dermatitis is one of the most common inflammatory skin diseases, affecting nearly **15% of children and 7% of adults worldwide**. To you, it feels like itchy, inflamed patches that refuse to go away. To me, it feels like chaos inside my microbial community. The disease is influenced by host genetics and the environment.

The Barrier That Breaks

Your skin barrier is your frontline defence. A key player here is a protein called **filaggrin** (a crucial component of the skin barrier) — it binds keratin fibres, helps maintain hydration, and keeps the skin strong.

But when **filaggrin is missing or defective**, your skin becomes leaky, dry, and weak. Its pH rises, creating a friendlier environment for unwanted guests like ***Staphylococcus aureus***. Without a strong wall, invaders march in, triggering immune alarms and inflammation.

My Microbial Shift in AD

When AD strikes, my usual diversity shrinks. Once-balanced microbial families are replaced by dominant troublemakers:

- **More of:**
  - *Staphylococcus aureus* → thrives in higher pH, produces toxins, and worsens inflammation.
  - *Staphylococcus epidermidis* → sometimes protective, but can also aggravate inflammation in excess.
- **Less of:**
  - *Cutibacterium spp.*→ normally helps with lipid metabolism.
  - *Corynebacterium spp.* and *Malassezia spp.* → usual residents that maintain equilibrium.

This **dysbiosis** leads to:

- The release of inflammatory cytokines (*signalling proteins that control inflammation*)
- The suppression of antimicrobial peptides (naturally occurring proteins that act as a first line of defence against a broad range of microbial threats)
- Disruption of lipid metabolism.

The result? The itchy, red, and dry patches you know as AD.

Skin and Gut: A Two-Way Conversation

You may think AD is only about your skin, but the story runs deeper. I am in constant conversation with your **gut microbiome**.

Not only the skin microbial dysbiosis but gut dysbiosis also plays a significant role in patients with atopic dermatitis. SCFAs (i.e., propionate, acetate, butyrate), end products of dietary fibre fermentation in your gut and are known to take an important part in shaping up the microbial composition and immune defence mechanism of the skin.

In AD, your gut microbiome and metabolome (the metabolites produced) are distinct as compared to healthy adults:

- **More of:** *Faecalibacterium prausnitzii, Clostridium spp., Escherichia spp.* → bacteria that damage gut lining and trigger inflammation.
- **Less of:** *Akkermansia, Bacteroidetes, Bifidobacterium* → protective microbes that calm the immune system.
- **Lower levels of SCFAs (butyrate, propionate, acetate):** these gut-fermented products normally reduce inflammation and help regulate immunity.

Microbial dysbiosis leads to a continuous inflammatory process in the gut.

When your gut is inflamed, your immune system stays on high alert. That inflammation reaches me, your skin, making AD worse.

Atopic dermatitis is associated with skin and gut microbial dysbiosis, selective modulation of the host flora to treat AD has become a centre of interest

Hidden Triggers of Atopic Dermatitis

1. **Vitamin D: More Than Just a Sunshine Vitamin**
    - Low vitamin D levels are linked with more severe cases of AD. Correcting this deficiency can significantly ease symptoms.
    - Vitamin D helps your skin's microbiome: it reduces the overgrowth of *Staphylococcus aureus* (a trouble-making bacterium) and encourages a healthier mix of microbes.
    - Beyond the skin, vitamin D also strengthens both the **gut and skin barriers**, keeping your body's defenses intact.

2. **Air Pollution: An Invisible Trigger**
   - Polluted air doesn't just harm your lungs — it can irritate your skin, too.
   - Tiny pollutants create **oxidative stress**, damaging skin cells and increasing the risk of AD flare-ups.
3. **Microbes and Early Life: Setting the Stage**
   - Your risk of developing AD can be shaped before you even say your first word.
   - Factors like **how you were delivered (C-section vs. natural birth)** and whether you have **siblings** influence your microbial "starter pack."
   - These early microbial differences may tip the balance toward — or away from — atopic dermatitis later in life.
   - **The Early Life Window** : Scientists also tell us that the seeds of AD are sown early. Babies with disrupted microbial colonization in their first months may develop an immune system skewed towards overreaction. This early imbalance sets the stage for AD later in life.

How Atopic Dermatitis Appears – Clinical Features

When the barrier is broken and I, your skin microbiome, lose balance, the changes become visible and hard to ignore. AD does not look the same in everyone — but here are the common features:

- **Itching (Pruritus):** the hallmark symptom, often worse at night, leading to scratching and further barrier damage.
- **Dry skin (Xerosis):** the skin cannot hold moisture, appearing rough and scaly.
- **Red, inflamed patches:** erythematous lesions often on the face, neck, hands, and flexural areas (elbows, knees).
- **Oozing and crusting:** in acute flares, especially when *Staphylococcus aureus* overgrows.

- **Thickened skin (Lichenification):** chronic scratching leads to thick, leathery patches.
- **Age-specific distribution:**
  - Infants → cheeks, scalp, extensor surfaces.
  - Children → flexural folds.
  - Adults → hands, eyelids, and flexures.

Every flare is a reflection of barrier dysfunction + microbial imbalance + immune overreaction.

Can Balance Be Restored?

The treatment of AD focuses on three goals:

1. **Repairing the barrier** → moisturizers and emollients.
2. **Reducing inflammation** → corticosteroids, calcineurin inhibitors.
3. **Reducing microbial overload** → antimicrobials and anti-staphylococcal therapies.

But scientists are now exploring deeper — targeting not just the skin, but also the **gut-skin axis**.

Treatment – Restoring Balance with Microbiome in Mind

Traditional treatment has focused on calming inflammation and repairing the barrier. But now, with me — your skin microbiome — in focus, newer approaches aim to **rebalance our microbial world**.

1. **Barrier Repair**
   - **Moisturizers & emollients**: restore hydration and strengthen the physical barrier.
   - **Ceramide-containing creams**: replace missing lipids that protect against microbial invasion and support growth of healthy commensals.

2. **Controlling Inflammation**
   - **Topical corticosteroids**: reduce cytokine storms and calm itching.
   - **Calcineurin inhibitors (Tacrolimus, Pimecrolimus)**: suppress local immune overreaction without thinning the skin.

3. **Antimicrobial Strategies**
   - **Targeting *Staphylococcus aureus* overgrowth**:
   - Bleach baths, topical antiseptics, or antibiotics during acute flares.
   - Narrow-spectrum therapies under study, to kill pathogens without harming protective microbes.

4. **Microbiome-Modulating Therapies**
   This is where science is evolving rapidly:
   - **Probiotics (oral):** *Lactobacillus* and *Bifidobacterium* strains reduce inflammation, improve barrier function, and enhance production of anti-inflammatory SCFAs in the gut.
   - **Topical probiotics:** creams containing beneficial bacteria or bacterial lysates aim to outcompete *S. aureus* and restore balance on the skin.
   - **Prebiotics (dietary fibers):** feed beneficial gut microbes, increasing SCFA production, which indirectly improves skin immunity.
   - **Synbiotics:** combining both pro- and prebiotics for stronger effects.
   - **Postbiotics (microbial metabolites):** topical or systemic use of SCFAs or bacterial-derived molecules to calm inflammation and support barrier repair.

POPULAR PROBIOTIC USED FOR GUT AND SKIN MICROBIOME ALTERATION

Lactobacillus spp.	*Bifidobacterium spp.*
Accelerate skin barrier recovery	Antipruritic effects (relieves itching) and anti-inflammatory
Anti-inflammatory- inhibits skin inflammation related to substance P	Antinociceptive (reducing perception of pain)

5. **Diet & Gut-Skin Axis**

   ○ Diets rich in **fiber, omega-3 fatty acids, and vitamins (D, B complex, zinc)** help reduce inflammation.

   ○ Avoiding **high-sugar and processed fats** lowers imbalanced sebum production and gut dysbiosis.

The future of AD therapy

Scientists are developing **live biotherapeutic products** — genetically engineered bacteria that live on your skin and produce anti-inflammatory molecules or antimicrobial peptides, directly at the site of imbalance. Early trials with **transplanting beneficial skin microbes** (like *Roseomonas mucosa*) have shown encouraging results in reducing disease severity.

Food items Recommended in individuals with Atopic dermatitis	Sources
Omega-3 Fatty Acids	Salmon, rohu, tuna, albacore, walnuts, flaxseeds, and chia seeds.
Antioxidants (Vitamin A, C, E)	Fruits (apples, blueberries, cherries, berries) and vegetables (spinach, kale).
Vitamin C-rich Foods	Bell peppers, oranges, strawberries, cauliflower, pineapple, and mangoes
Nuts and Seeds	Brazil nuts and flaxseeds
Whole Grains	Wheat, oats, buckwheat
Probiotics	Yogurt, kimchi, sauerkraut, and other fermented foods
Potassium-rich Foods:	Bananas, sweet potatoes, spinach.

Reducing lesion severity, Reduce skin inflammation, Decrease dryness and itching

To reduce the oxidative stress, the major pathological change in patients with AD

Brazilian nut - Good antioxidant property , high protein value; Flax seeds – good source of omega 3 fatty acids and high fibre content

Anti-inflammatory properties, maintain hydration of skin

Maintain healthy gut microbiome

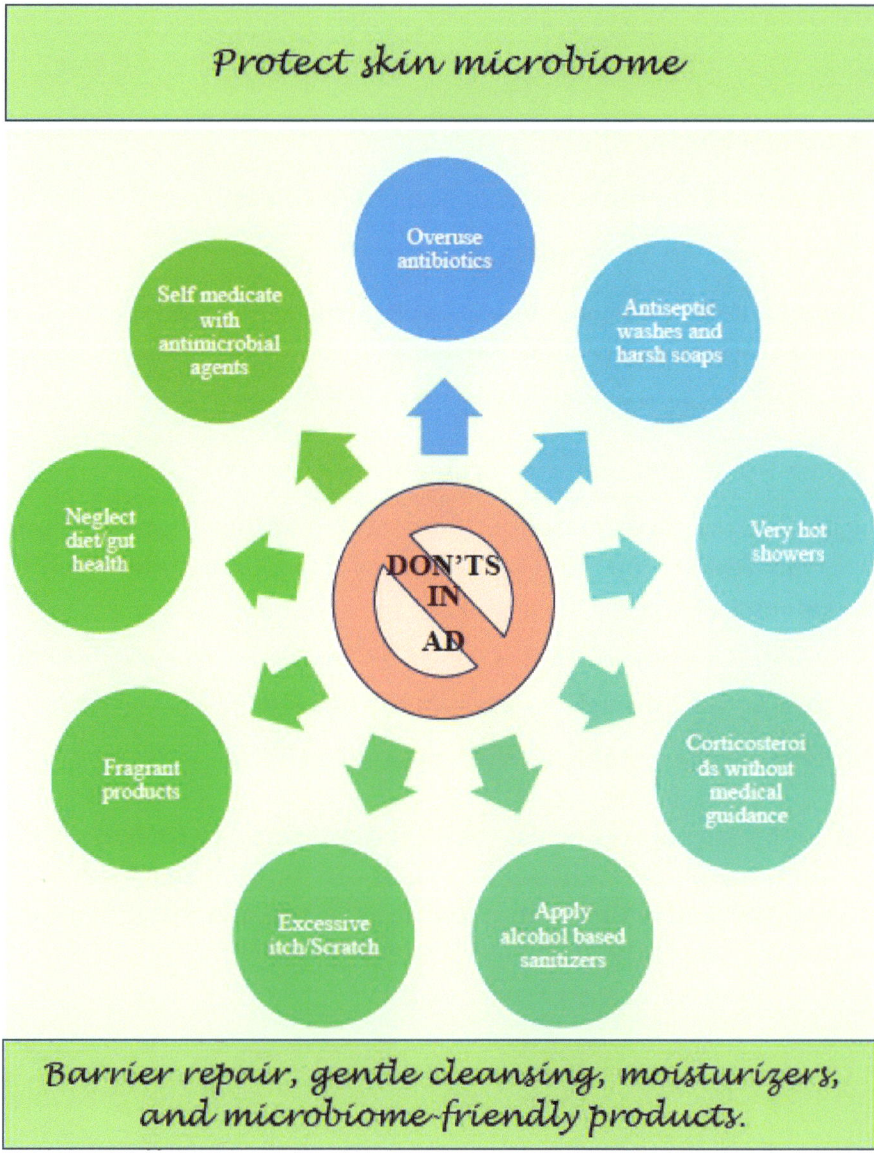
Protect skin microbiome
Overuse antibiotics
Antiseptic washes and harsh soaps
Very hot showers
Corticosteroids without medical guidance
Apply alcohol based sanitizers
Excessive itch/Scratch
Fragrant products
Neglect diet/gut health
Self medicate with antimicrobial agents
DON'TS IN AD
Barrier repair, gentle cleansing, moisturizers, and microbiome-friendly products.

Key Message

Atopic Dermatitis is not just an itchy rash — it is a **triangular story** of:

- A **broken barrier** (filaggrin deficiency),
- A **disturbed microbiome** (skin and gut dysbiosis),
- And an **overactive immune system** (inflammatory cascades).
- Treatment is no longer only about creams and steroids — it is about **restoring microbial harmony** on both skin and gut. When my world regains balance, your skin regains peace.

6. **Probiotics, Prebiotics, and Synbiotics**
   - **Probiotics (live beneficial bacteria like** ***Lactobacillus*** **and** ***Bifidobacterium*****) help rebalance the gut and soothe inflammation.**
   - **Prebiotics (fibers that feed good bacteria) increase SCFA production, strengthening immune tolerance.**
   - **Synbiotics combine both for enhanced effect.**

When ingested, probiotics can shape gut flora, calm inflammation, and indirectly benefit me, your skin. When applied topically, they can even help reorganize my community directly at the skin level.

"I am your skin microbiome, your invisible guardian. When your barrier is strong and my community is diverse, your skin feels calm and whole. But when filaggrin is lost, when ***Staphylococcus*** **dominates, and when your gut no longer speaks in harmony with me, I falter — and you feel the flare. Care for me with moisture, nourishment, and microbial support, and together we can quiet the itch and heal the skin."**

Chapter 7
Psoriasis
My plaque look

My Life in Diseased Skin

I am your **skin microbiome** — your invisible community of guardians. I usually live in harmony with you, balancing invaders and training your immune system. But in psoriasis, my world is disrupted.

Instead of calm coexistence, I watch **keratinocytes grow uncontrollably**, piling into **thick, scaly plaques**. Your skin barrier weakens, and your immune system turns hyperactive. What you see as the **itchy, red, silvery patches**, I feel as **a battlefield filled with chaos**.

Your **genes, lifestyle, and environment** all pull the strings of this chronic inflammatory drama.

Clinical Features – What Psoriasis Looks Like from My Side

When I lose balance, the changes in your skin are striking:

- **Sharp, red plaques with silvery scales** — my most visible distress signal.
- **Itching (pruritus)** — you scratch, tearing the barrier further and worsening my imbalance.
- **Auspitz sign** — tiny bleeding spots when scales are scraped off, evidence of how fragile the barrier has become.
- **Koebner phenomenon** — new lesions appear where your skin is injured, reminding me how vulnerable I've become.
- **Different faces of the disease**:
    - **Plaque psoriasis**: the classic form, on scalp, elbows, knees.
    - **Guttate psoriasis**: small drop-like spots, often after a *Streptococcus* infection.

  - **Inverse psoriasis**: shiny red lesions in folds.
  - **Pustular psoriasis**: sterile pustules forming on inflamed skin.
  - **Erythrodermic psoriasis**: widespread redness, dangerously destabilizing your body.
- **Nails join in** — pitting, yellow "oil-drop" discoloration, and crumbling edges.
- **Joints ache** — in psoriatic arthritis, inflammation spreads deeper, stiffening your movements.

Every symptom is a reflection of **barrier disruption, immune overreaction, and my altered microbial composition**.

My Altered Skin Microbial World

In healthy skin, I — your microbiome — am diverse, balanced, and protective. But psoriasis pushes me into disorder:

- **More of my aggressive residents**: *Staphylococcus* and *Streptococcus* species rise in numbers.
- **Fewer of my protectors**: *Staphylococcus epidermidis* and *Cutibacterium acnes* decline, making it easier for *S. aureus* to take over.

This imbalance amplifies inflammation and fuels the chronic cycle of disease.

The Gut–Skin Conversation in Psoriasis

I'm not alone in this struggle. My distant cousin — your **gut microbiome** — is also disrupted in psoriasis.

- **Fewer of the peacekeepers**: *Bacteroidetes*, *Faecalibacterium*, *Akkermansia muciniphila*, *Lachnospira*.
- **More of the troublemakers**: *Firmicutes* like *Ruminococcus torques* and *R. gnavus*.

When the gut barrier weakens, harmful metabolites and antigens leak into your blood. This keeps your immune system on high alert, intensifying inflammation that eventually reaches me, your skin.

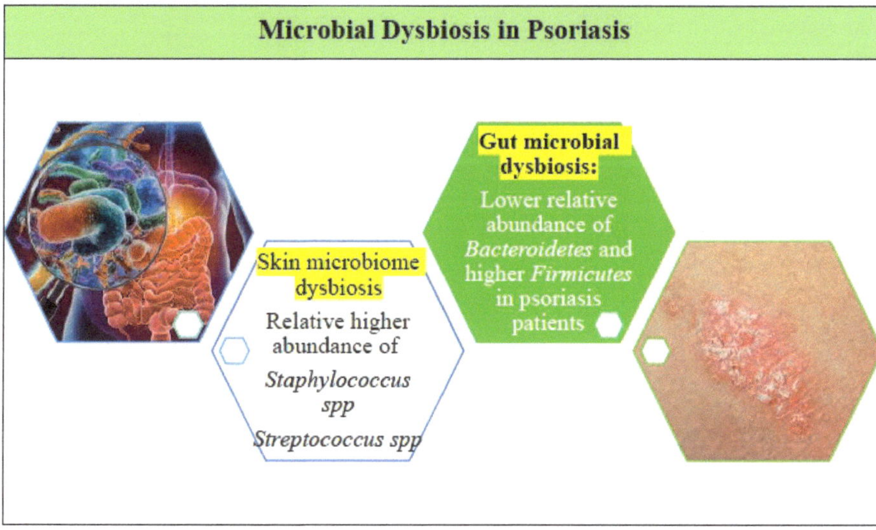

That is why psoriasis is not just a **skin disease**, but a **systemic inflammatory condition**, linked with **IBD, celiac disease, obesity, and metabolic syndrome**.

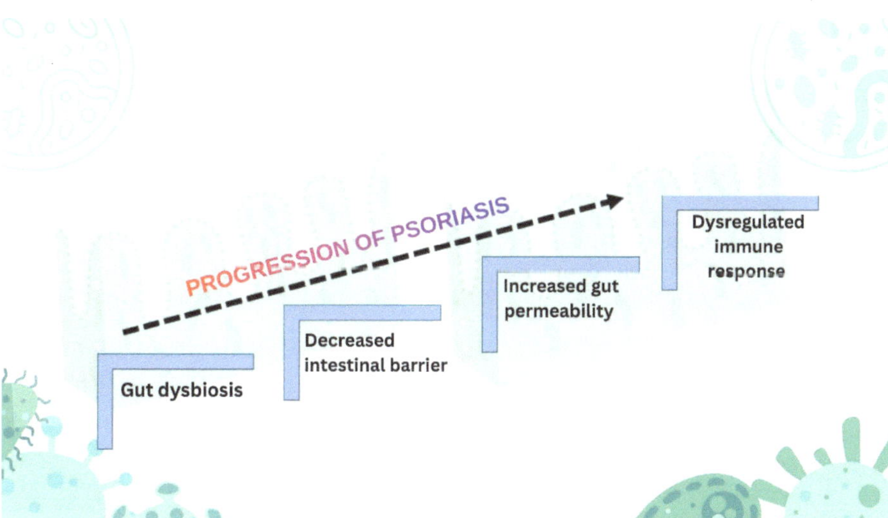

Hidden Triggers I Face

- **Infections:** A *Streptococcus* throat infection often unleashes guttate psoriasis, worsening my imbalance.
- **Lactose intolerance:** more common in people with psoriasis, tied to increased disease severity.
- **Environmental stressors:** air pollution, high-fat diets, stress, and alcohol all disturb both me and your gut microbes.

Amazing Facts from My Perspective

1. People with psoriasis have higher risk of gut immune diseases (IBD, UC, celiac).
2. Lactose intolerance is more common and linked with worse psoriasis.
3. Guttate psoriasis often follows a *Streptococcus* throat infection — some even need tonsil removal.
4. Treatments that target inflammation also shift my microbial balance, sometimes restoring diversity.
5. Probiotics are showing promise — when given to psoriasis patients, they lower relapses and calm systemic inflammation.

How Treatments Change My World

For years, treatment focused on suppressing your immune system and calming skin flares. But I can tell you — therapies also reshape me, the microbiome.

1. **Conventional approaches**
    - **Topical corticosteroids and vitamin D analogues** calm inflammation and reduce scaling.
    - **Methotrexate, cyclosporin, retinoids, fumarates** work deeper, modulating immunity across your body.
    - **Biologics** (adalimumab, ustekinumab, secukinumab, ixekizumab) target cytokines like TNF-⍰, IL-12/23, IL-17 — they

help me indirectly by reducing inflammation that drives microbial imbalance.

2. **Microbiome-targeted approaches**

   ○ **Narrowband UVB therapy**: trims down pathogenic *Staphylococcus* and *Firmicutes*, giving space for protective microbes to recover.

   ○ **Systemics and biologics**: alter gut microbiome balance (Actinobacteria:Firmicutes ratio), with biologics showing the strongest effect.

   ○ **Probiotics**: adding *Lactobacillus* and *Bifidobacterium* strains improves gut health, reduces relapses, and indirectly helps me restore balance.

3. **Diet and lifestyle**

- **High-fat diets worsen me** — they increase systemic inflammation and microbial imbalance.
- **Balanced fibre-rich diets** encourage SCFA production, calming inflammation and supporting both gut and skin harmony.
- **Restricted FODMAP (Fermentable oligosaccharides, disaccharides, monosaccharides and polyols) is the key to achieving calm in psoriasis.**
- **Low FODMAP diet includes:**
  - ○ **Fruits: grapes, strawberries, oranges, kiwi**
  - ○ **Vegetables: carrot, spinach, cucumber**
  - ○ **Grains: oats (avoid gluten)**
  - ○ **Dairy alternatives: oat milk, cheese**

Omega 3 fatty acids

Fish (salmon, mackerel, and tuna) nuts and seeds (walnuts, chia seeds, and flaxseeds)

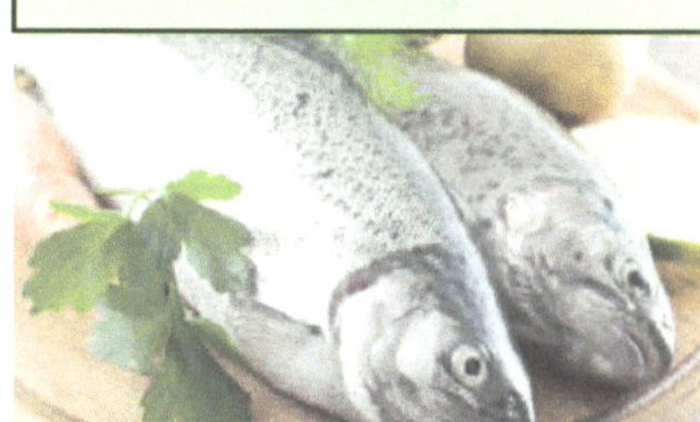

1. Improved metabolic profile
2. Increased responsiveness to immunomodulating treatment.
3. Alters gut microbiota influencing decreased release of pro-inflammatory cytokines.

- **Omega 3 rich diet**
  - **High-quality proteins from lean sources**
    - **Salmon, tuna, mackerel**
  - **Plant-based foods**
    - **Nuts and seeds**

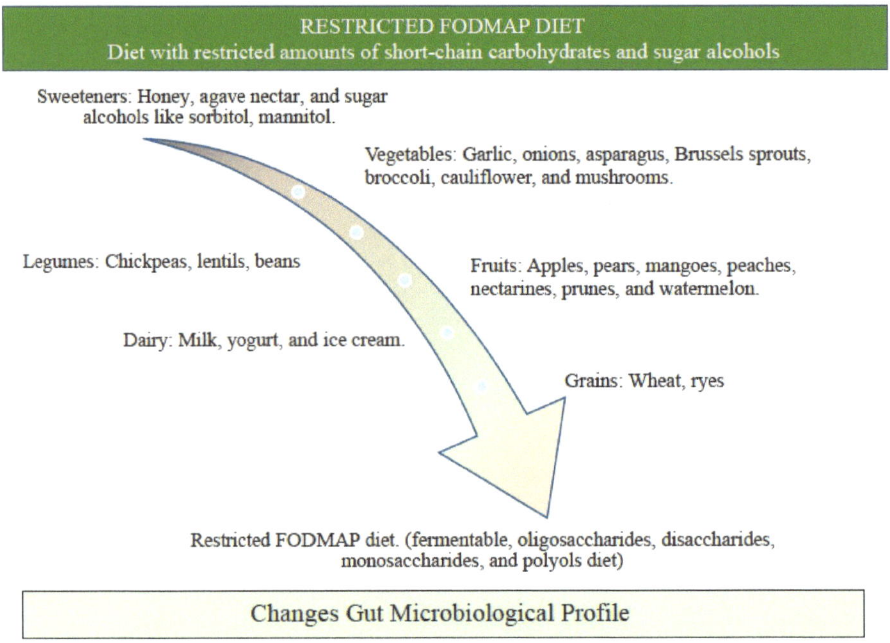

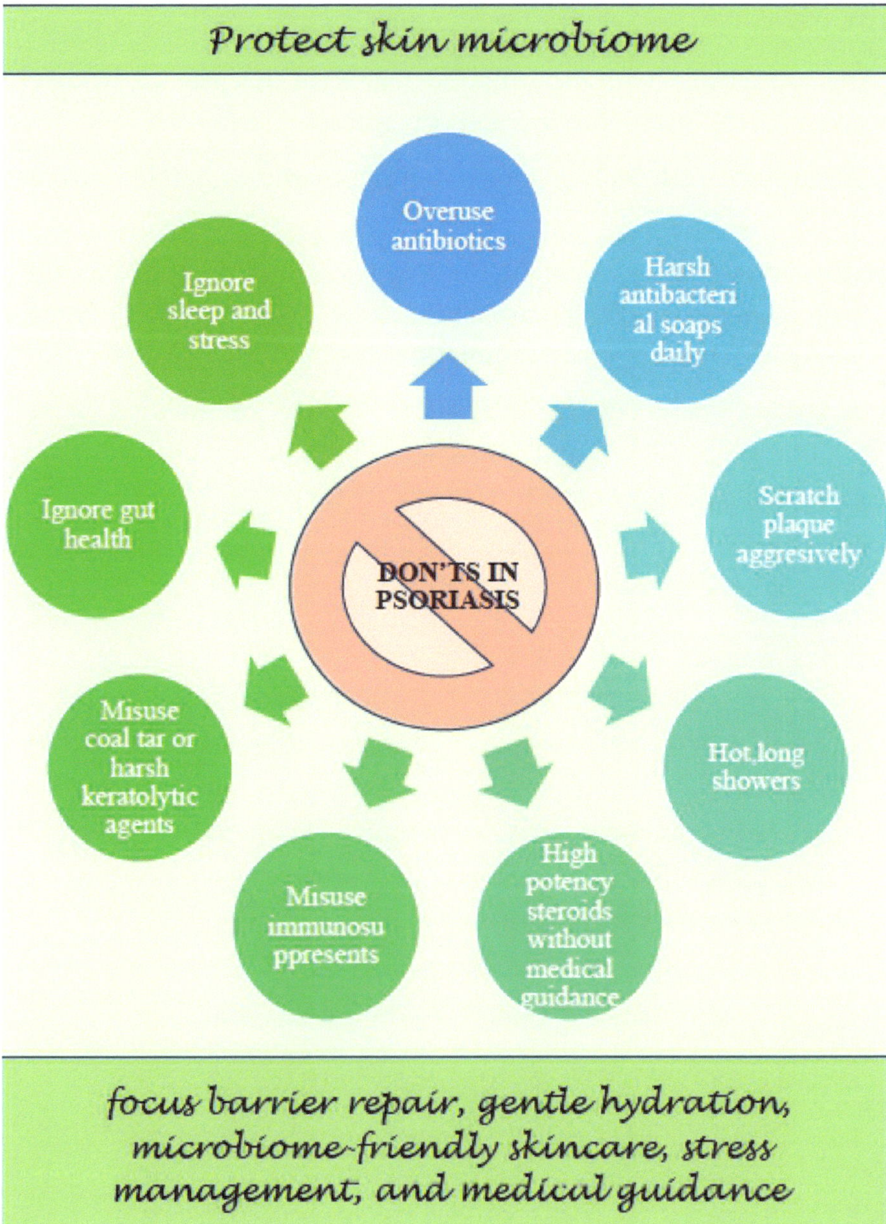
Protect skin microbiome
Overuse antibiotics
Harsh antibacterial soaps daily
Scratch plaque aggresively
Hot,long showers
High potency steroids without medical guidance
Misuse immunosuppresents
Misuse coal tar or harsh keratolytic agents
Ignore gut health
Ignore sleep and stress
DON'TS IN PSORIASIS
focus barrier repair, gentle hydration, microbiome-friendly skincare, stress management, and medical guidance

Key Message:

1. **Disease Basics:** Chronic inflammatory skin disease; keratinocyte overgrowth, immune hyperactivity, microbial imbalance.
2. **Symptoms:** Red, scaly plaques; itching; fragile skin; nail and joint involvement.
3. **Microbiome Imbalance:** Aggressive bacteria ↑ (Staphylococcus, Streptococcus), protective bacteria ↓ (S. epidermidis, C. acnes); gut dysbiosis worsens inflammation.
4. **Triggers:** Streptococcus infections, lactose intolerance, stress, high-fat diet, alcohol, pollution.
5. **Management:** Treatments (topicals, systemic drugs, biologics), microbiome-targeted approaches (UVB, probiotics), and lifestyle/diet changes restore balance and reduce flares.

"I am your skin microbiome, your hidden ecosystem. When psoriasis takes hold, I change — diversity shrinks, pathogens rise, and your skin barrier collapses into chronic inflammation. Care for me — through balanced diet, probiotics, barrier repair, and mindful treatments — and I can help restore harmony. When your gut and skin speak in unity, psoriasis flares can soften, and together we can move toward calm, healthy skin."

Chapter 8
Dandruff
My white flaky home

Your **scalp microbiome**, resides in a unique neighbourhood—the scalp. Most of the time, we keep everything balanced. But when harmony is disturbed, **dandruff** appears. Dandruff, the flaky scalp, a skin condition of your scalp associated with pruritis. Occurs in 30-50% of the world's population. Males are generally more affected than females. A severe form of dandruff involving chronic inflammation of the skin with recurrent character is known as seborrheic dermatitis.

My Favourite Home: The Hair Follicle

My favourite place to live is the **hair follicle**. Follicles are not just hair factories — they are **microbial habitats**.

- **Sebaceous glands** that release lipid-rich sebum, my primary energy source.
- **Sweat glands** that alter pH and moisture
- **Hair shafts** are tiny microenvironments where different microbes thrive.

Your hair follicle is home to a **complex microbial ecosystem**, including bacteria, fungi, viruses, and archaea. Together, these create **distinct niches** where different microbes thrive. Most of the time, we live peacefully, keeping your scalp healthy.

My Role in Your Scalp Health

I am not just a bystander — I actively influence your scalp:

- I **support hair growth cycles** by interacting with follicular cells.
- I **modulate stress responses**, helping your skin remain resilient when you're under pressure.
- I **protect against invaders**, preventing colonization by harmful microbes.

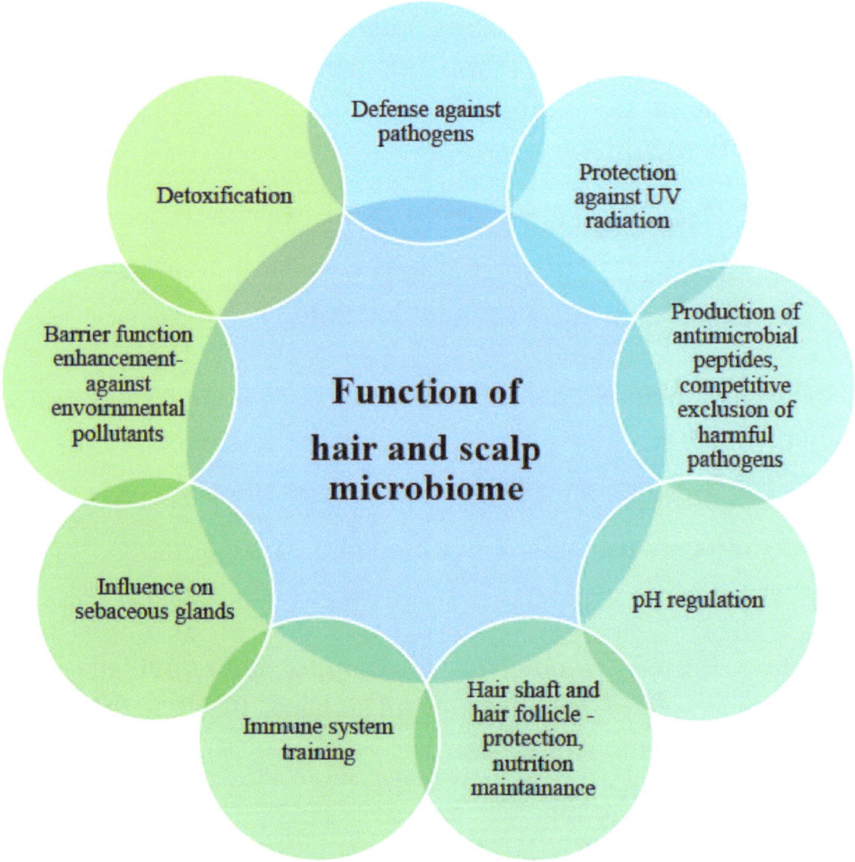

Bacterial residents include: These bacteria help maintain follicle health by modulating stress responses and preventing harmful pathogens from taking over.

- *Cutibacterium (Propionibacterium) acnes*- helps metabolize sebum.
- *Staphylococcus epidermidis* acts like a guardian, producing antimicrobial peptides
- *Corynebacterium spp. maintains the final equilibrium*

Fungal residents include:

- *Malassezia* species especially *M. restricta* and *M. globosa*, dominate in oily regions — but if they grow unchecked, they trigger irritation and inflammation.
- Yeasts, are **lipophilic (oil-loving)** and thrive in sebaceous areas such as the scalp, face, ears, and upper trunk

Predominance of fungal organisms on the scalp, particularly *Malassezia* species, triggers an inflammatory response that manifests clinically as dandruff or seborrheic dermatitis. Because *Malassezia* is a lipophilic (lipid-loving) fungus, it preferentially colonizes areas rich in sebaceous glands—such as the scalp, face, ears, and upper trunk. Individuals with oily skin are therefore more susceptible to seborrheic dermatitis. Dominated scalp microbiome includes *Malassezia* species (*M. restricta, M. globosa, M. furfur*). Abundance of *Malassezia spp.* leads to overproduction of oleic acid and other irritant free fatty acids in the scalp microenvironment.

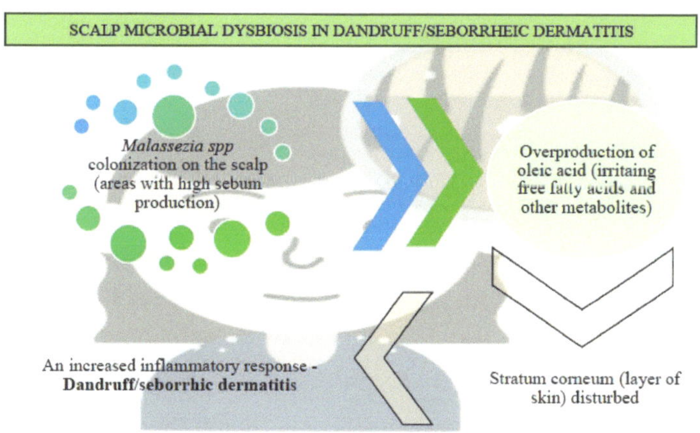

This shift leads to **inflammation, itching, and visible flaking**.

> Your hair follicle is more than just a root of your hair — it is a **living microbial ecosystem**, with me as its caretaker. As long as harmony is preserved, I keep your scalp healthy and comfortable. But if my world is disrupted… that's when the white flakes start to appear.
>
> - *Malassezia* species become **overabundant**
> - Protective bacteria like *Staphylococcus* may **decline**
> - *Cutibacterium acnes* may increase, disrupting lipid metabolism

Why Balance Breaks

Like many other skin conditions, **dandruff is multifactorial**. Whether I stay balanced or fall into chaos depends on many things:

- The **sebum** your sebaceous glands produce (too much oil feeds certain fungi, too little destabilizes my balance).
- The strength of your **immune system** (sometimes it overreacts to harmless microbes).
- **Stress and hormones**, which change both oil production and microbial activity.
- **Environmental influences**, such as humidity, pollution, or harsh hair products.
- And of course, your **individual genetic sensitivity**. Some scalps simply react more strongly than others.

Scientists are still unravelling the exact cause of dandruff, but they agree that **my microbial balance plays a central role**.

How Dandruff/Seborrheic Dermatitis presents clinically

When your scalp microbiome falls out of balance, dandruff reveals itself through a mix of visible and sensory signs:

- **Flakes**: White or yellowish, loose flakes on the scalp, hair, or shoulders
- **Itching**: Persistent scalp itch, sometimes accompanied by tingling or burning
- **Dryness or greasiness**: Depending on sebum levels, the scalp may feel unusually dry or oily
- **Redness and irritation**: Inflamed scalp patches in moderate to severe cases
- **Scaling**: Fine scaling in mild cases, thicker or greasy scales in seborrheic dermatitis
- **Chronic course**: Symptoms often come and go in cycles of shedding and regrowth

The Gut–Skin Connection

You may think dandruff begins and ends on the scalp — but my story reaches deeper, into your **gut**. Scientists have detected subtle **deviations in the intestinal mucosa** of patients with seborrheic dermatitis, suggesting that your gut and scalp might be more connected than you realize.

Still, the link between **gut dysbiosis** (an imbalance of intestinal microbes) and dandruff remains **controversial**. Some studies suggest a connection, others don't. But here's what we know for sure: your **diet directly influences sebum production**.

- **Dietary lipids, glucose, and acetate** stimulate sebaceous gland activity.
- **High sugar intake** is commonly seen in individuals with seborrheic dermatitis.
- Restricting **calorie-dense, sugary, or fatty foods** is associated with lower sebum production.

This is why people with dandruff are often advised to:

- Avoid sugar, animal fats and greasy fried foods
- Increase vegetables, water-rich fruits, seeds, fish, biotin, and vitamin B

Although these dietary recommendations sound convincing, the **scientific evidence remains inconclusive**.

Can Probiotics Help?

Since microbial imbalance plays such a big role in dandruff, researchers have explored ways to **restore balance using probiotics**. Both **oral and topical probiotic formulations** have been tested.

One **clinical study** using *Lactobacillus paracasei* showed **significant improvement in dandruff severity and symptoms** in patients with moderate to severe cases. This suggests that supporting your **gut and scalp microbiome together** may be a promising path for future treatment.

Probiotics and dandruff •*L. paracasei* •*L. plantarum* •*B. lactis*	Include specific strains of bacteria and fungi	•Restore microbial balance by inhibiting the growth of dandruff-causing fungi *Malassezia spp.*
	•Produce antimicrobial peptides and metabolites	•Restore healthier microbial niche on the scalp.
	•Enhance production of ceramides, play a crucial role in maintaining the scalp's moisture balance	•This helps prevent dryness, flaking, and itching associated with dandruff
	•Modulate immune response	•Regulating excessive production of sebum
	•Produce antimicrobial compounds with antagonistic activity against dandruff-causing pathogens. Compounds, such as bacilysin and bacillomycin D	•Inhibit the growth of *Malassezia* species biofilms (fungal colonies).

Restoring Balance

Treatment focuses on microbial balance, inflammation control, and skin barrier support:

Topical Therapies

- Anti-fungal shampoos (ketoconazole, zinc pyrithione)
- Corticosteroid lotions for inflammation
- Gentle scalp care routines
- Essential oils of herbal origin, such as tea tree oil, lime oil and rosemary oil, have gained global importance in hair care. These oils are rich in aromatic secondary metabolites, especially terpenes and phenolic components that impart substantial antimicrobial properties and help resist biofilm formation

Systemic Approaches

- Oral antifungals in resistant cases
- Nutritional support: vitamins B, D, zinc, omega-3 fatty acids

Microbiome Support

- Prebiotic or probiotic formulations for scalp health
- Stress management and gentle hair care

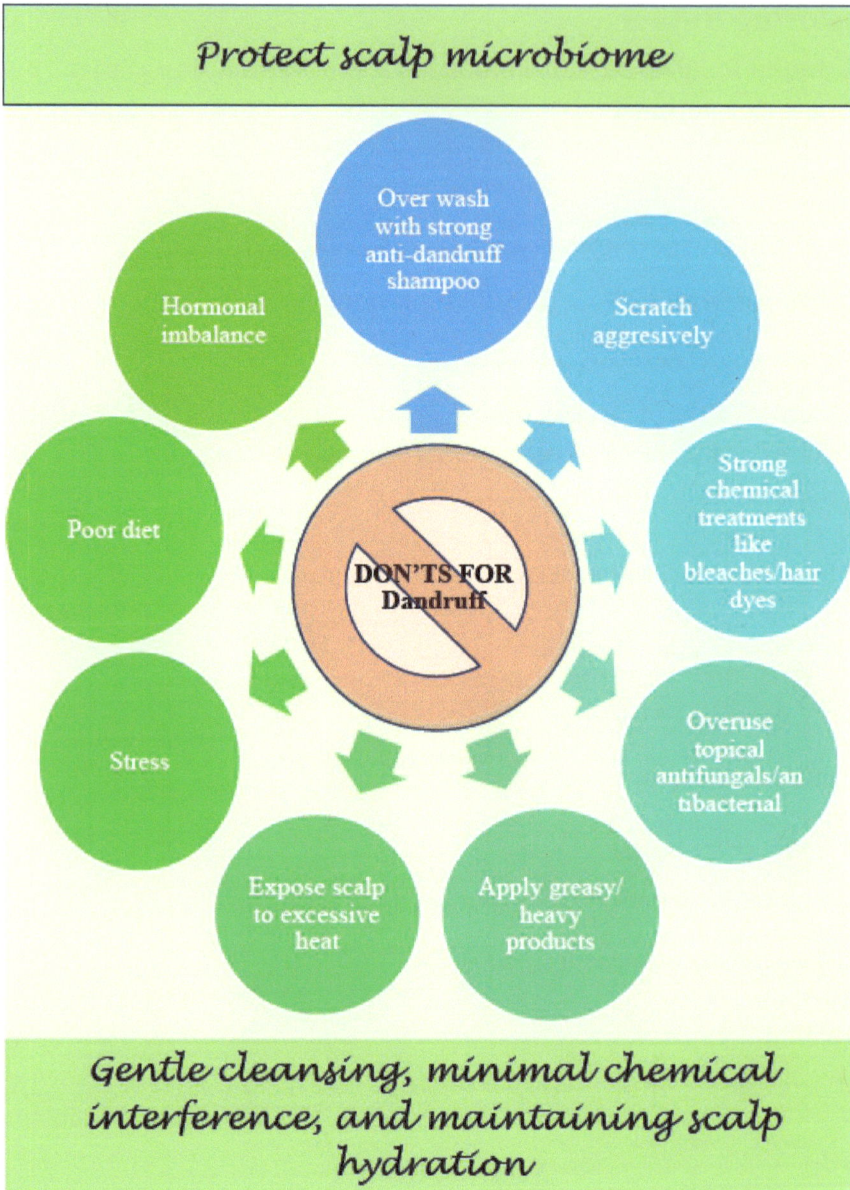
Protect scalp microbiome
Over wash with strong anti-dandruff shampoo
Scratch aggresively
Strong chemical treatments like bleaches/hair dyes
Overuse topical antifungals/an tibacterial
Apply greasy/ heavy products
Expose scalp to excessive heat
Stress
Poor diet
Hormonal imbalance
DON'TS FOR Dandruff
Gentle cleansing, minimal chemical interference, and maintaining scalp hydration

Key Messages

- **Dandruff and seborrheic dermatitis** affect 30–50% of the global population, with males more commonly affected.
- The condition is **multifactorial**, involving sebum production, microbial imbalance (especially *Malassezia* spp.), immune responses, stress, hormones, and environmental factors.
- **Scalp microbiome dysbiosis** — overgrowth of *Malassezia* with altered *Staphylococcus* and *Cutibacterium* populations — plays a central role in disease development.
- **Gut–skin axis** and dietary habits may influence dandruff severity, though evidence remains inconclusive.
- **Treatment strategies** focus on antifungal agents, anti-inflammatory therapies, barrier repair, and microbiome modulation (e.g., probiotics).

"I am your scalp microbiome — when harmony is kept, I protect, nourish, and comfort you. But when my balance is lost, the white flakes begin to fall. Care for me gently, and I will keep your scalp a healthy home."

Chapter 9

Rosacea

My angry red look

A Fiery Conversation Between Us

I am your skin microbiome, the community of tiny protectors that live with you every day. Usually, I help keep peace on your face — balancing inflammation, training immunity, and holding off invaders. But in rosacea, this balance falters. Your skin becomes flushed, red, and sometimes bumpy, while I struggle with overgrowth and dysregulation inside my world.

How Rosacea Appears – The Clinical Face

When I am disturbed, your skin shows it clearly:

- **Redness and flushing** that often worsens with triggers like alcohol, hot drinks, or spicy food.
- **Visible blood vessels (telangiectasia)** crossing cheeks and nose.
- **Papulopustular lesion** — acne-like spots filled with pus.
- **Ocular rosacea** in some of you, causing burning of eyes, irritation, and even corneal problems.
- A background of **sensitive, burning skin** that reacts easily to sun, temperature, or cosmetics.

Why This Happens – Immune & Barrier Chaos

The reason I lose control lies deeper:

- Your **innate immune system** becomes overactive, releasing abnormal levels of inflammatory cytokines.

- **Cathelicidins**, normally protective antimicrobial peptides, are overproduced — but in altered forms that drive inflammation instead of calming it.
- Your blood vessels overreact to signals, leading to **neurovascular dysregulation** — the flushes and persistent redness you see.
- Genes and environment play important role: fair skin, UV radiation, stress, and irritant exposures all push me into imbalance.

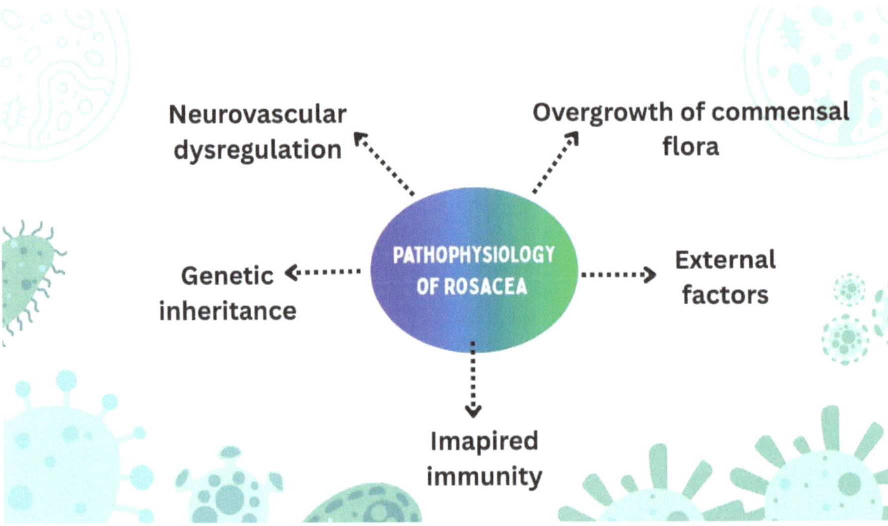

My Shifting Composition in Rosacea

In rosacea, my family of microbes changes dramatically:

- **More of**:
  - *Demodex folliculorum* (mites) — taking shelter in your sebaceous glands.
  - *Staphylococcus epidermidis* and *Bacillus oleronius* — bacteria that inflame and irritate.
  - *Cutibacterium acnes* — sometimes helpful, but disruptive in excess.
- **Less balance overall**: instead of harmony, certain members dominate, driving inflammation.

- Scientists tried removing *Demodex* with mite-killing creams. The mites decreased, but the skin lesions remained — proving it's not just one culprit, but the whole microbial and immune orchestra gone wrong.

The Gut–Skin Conversation

I don't live alone on your face; I talk constantly with your gut microbes. In rosacea, they too are disturbed:

- Less microbial diversity, and more of *Acidaminococcus* and *Megasphaera*.
- Fewer protective groups like *Peptococcaceae* and *Methanobrevibacter*.
- Many rosacea patients harbor ***Helicobacter pylori*** **infection**, causing gastritis and acid reflux.
- Others show **SIBO (small intestinal bacterial overgrowth)** — when treated, their facial redness and bumps often improve.

Your gut and I share signals. When it is inflamed, those messages reach me, worsening your rosacea.

Triggers and Daily Life

I flare when you expose me to:

- Hot drinks, alcohol, spicy foods, cinnamon-rich foods.
- Heat and sunlight.
- Stress and emotional surges.

But I calm down when you follow an **anti-inflammatory, Mediterranean-style diet** — fruits, vegetables, oily fishes, nuts, seeds — and avoid the known triggers.

Amazing Facts I Hold

1. If you live with rosacea, you're more likely to also have **gastric problems** like reflux or IBD.
2. Treating **H. pylori infection** or **SIBO** can sometimes improve rosacea symptoms.
3. My imbalance is not just on your face — it reflects your whole body's microbial and immune health.
4. Lifestyle and diet are as powerful as creams or pills in calming the disease.

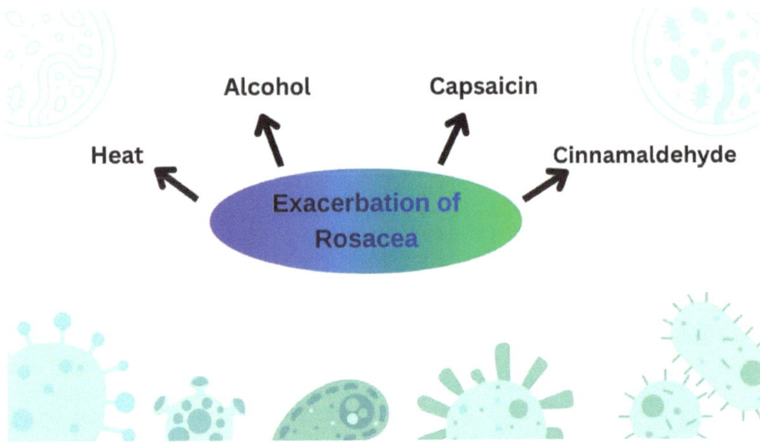

Treatment – Restoring Balance With Me in Mind

The goal of rosacea treatment is not just to mask the redness but to calm inflammation, repair your barrier, and rebalance your microbiome.

1. **Controlling Inflammation & Flushing**
   - **Topical therapies**: metronidazole, azelaic acid, ivermectin (target mites & bacteria).
   - **Oral agents**: doxycycline (low-dose, anti-inflammatory), tetracycline.
   - **Vascular-targeted**: brimonidine gel and oxymetazoline reduce redness by constricting dilated vessels.

2. Microbial Strategies

- **Anti-mite therapies**: permethrin and ivermectin reduce *Demodex* load, though not always sufficient alone.
- **Antibiotics**: oral or topical to suppress *Staphylococcus* and *Bacillus* species during flares.
- **Probiotics (oral and topical)**: under study to rebalance both gut and skin microbiomes, potentially reducing flare severity.

3. Gut–Skin Axis Care

- Testing and treatment for ***H. pylori*** infection or **SIBO** may improve rosacea.
- Prebiotic and probiotic approaches may enhance microbial diversity, reducing inflammation.

4. Lifestyle & Diet

- **Avoid triggers**: alcohol, hot drinks, spicy foods, extreme heat.
- **Mediterranean diet**: rich in anti-inflammatory nutrients, protective for both gut and skin.
- **Stress management**: mindfulness and relaxation reduce flare frequency.

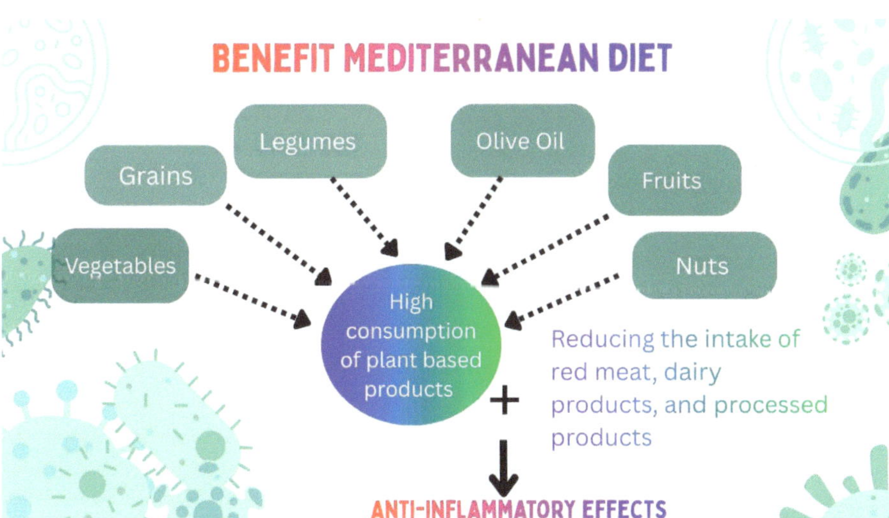

Future Therapies – Where Science is Heading

Researchers are beginning to see me not as a problem to be wiped away, but as a partner to be guided. In rosacea, the therapies of tomorrow may include:

- **Live biotherapeutic products**: beneficial bacteria designed to colonize your skin, producing anti-inflammatory molecules directly at the site of redness.
- **Topical microbiome transplants**: restoring missing protective microbes to crowd out harmful ones.
- **Postbiotics**: applying microbial metabolites — like short-chain fatty acids or bacterial peptides — to reduce inflammation and support barrier repair.
- **Precision probiotics**: oral strains tailored to reduce SIBO, improve gut balance, and send calming signals to me, your skin microbiome.

The future may shift from suppressing flares to **rebuilding harmony**, where my diversity is restored and your skin glows calm again.

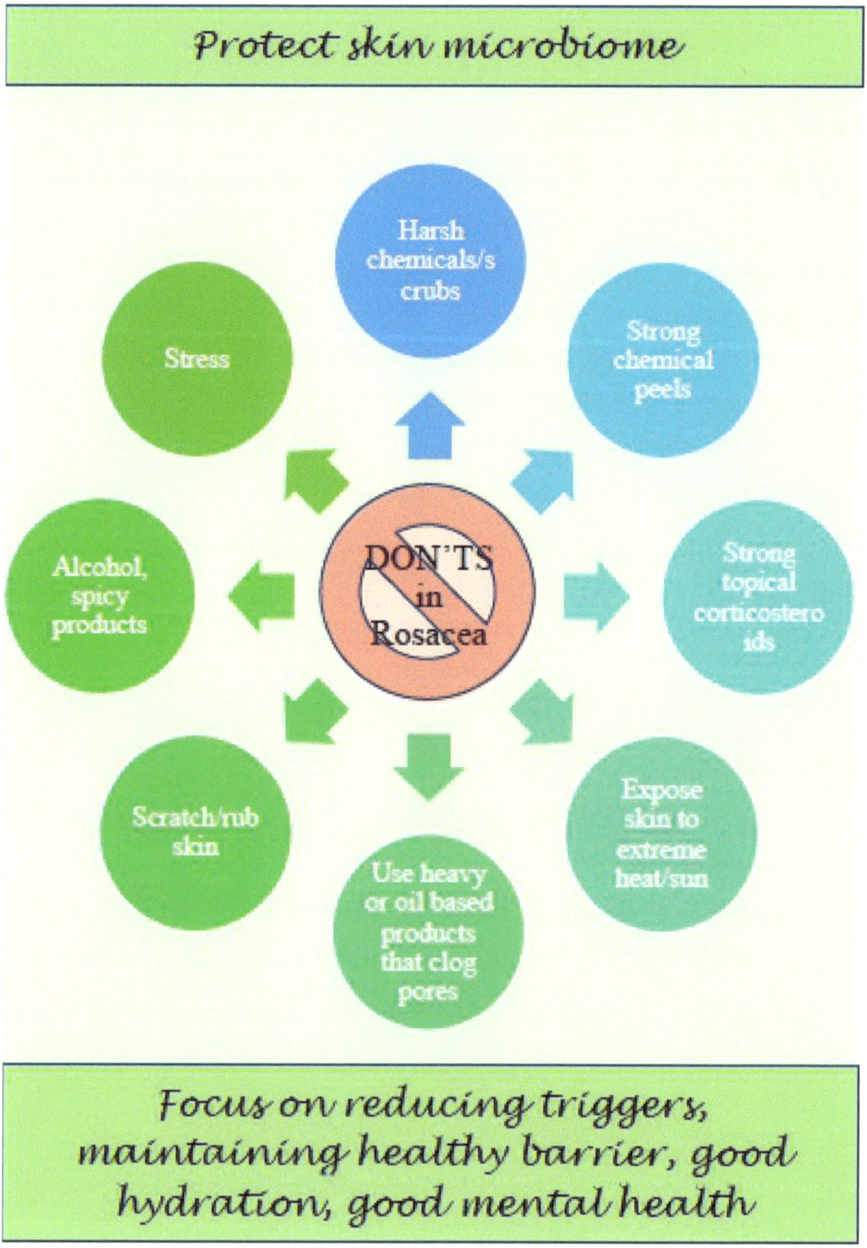
Protect skin microbiome
DON'TS in Rosacea
Harsh chemicals/scrubs
Strong chemical peels
Strong topical corticosteroids
Expose skin to extreme heat/sun
Use heavy or oil based products that clog pores
Scratch/rub skin
Alcohol, spicy products
Stress
Focus on reducing triggers, maintaining healthy barrier, good hydration, good mental health

Key Message

1. **Disease Basics:** Chronic inflammatory skin condition; microbiome imbalance drives redness, flushing, bumps, and irritation.
2. **Symptoms:** Facial redness, flushing, papulopustules, visible blood vessels, sensitive or burning skin, sometimes ocular involvement.
3. **Microbiome Changes:** Overgrowth of Demodex mites, *Staphylococcus epidermidis, Bacillus oleronius,* and *Cutibacterium acnes*; overall loss of microbial balance. Gut dysbiosis (H. pylori, SIBO) worsens inflammation.
4. **Triggers:** Hot drinks, alcohol, spicy foods, heat, sunlight, stress, and irritants.
5. **Management:** Anti-inflammatory topicals and oral agents, anti-mite therapies, probiotics, gut care, trigger avoidance, Mediterranean diet, and stress management. Future therapies focus on restoring microbial harmony.

"I am your skin microbiome. In rosacea, I tip out of balance — with mites, bacteria, and immune chaos all joining the storm. But when your gut is healthy, your diet calming, and your triggers avoided, I can regain harmony. Protect me, and I will protect the calmness of your face."

Chapter 10

Alopecia Areata

My Patchy Bald Look

Your scalp microbiome, usually thriving in balance across your scalp and hair follicles. Together, my microbial family and your immune system maintain the health of your hair and its roots. But sometimes, when my harmony is disturbed and your immune system turns against its own follicles, I manifest as **Alopecia Areata** — that sudden, patchy bald look that often feels like a nightmare.

Clinical presentation of my patchy bald look

Alopecia areata typically presents as **well-demarcated, round or oval patches of hair loss** on the scalp. In more severe cases, it may extend to involve the beard, eyebrows, eyelashes, or even the entire body. The affected skin often looks smooth and normal, without scaling or scarring, but the loss of hair is striking. Sometimes, "exclamation mark hairs" — short broken hairs tapering at the base — appear at the patch margins, serving as a clinical clue.

The Immune Chaos

At the root of this condition lies an **autoimmune attack** on the hair follicle. Normally, your hair follicle enjoys a state of "immune privilege," protecting it from inflammatory damage. But in alopecia areata, this privilege collapses.

- **Innate and adaptive immune cells** infiltrate the follicular environment.
- Elevated **cytokines** such as interferon-γ and interleukin-15 drive inflammation.
- The result: follicular cycling is disrupted, hair growth halts, and patches of baldness emerge.

Why this immune response gets triggered remains uncertain, but a combination of **genetic susceptibility**, **environmental stressors**, and **microbial imbalance** contributes to the disease onset.

The Scalp Microbiome Connection

On your healthy scalp, I — your microbiome — am mainly composed of ***Corynebacteriaceae*, *Propionibacteriaceae* (*Cutibacterium*), and *Staphylococcaceae***. A small but significant part of me is fungal, with ***Malassezia restricta*** dominating. When balanced, we coexist peacefully. But in alopecia areata, my composition shifts:

- **Increased *Cutibacterium acnes*** with a **decrease in *Staphylococcus epidermidis*** create dysbiosis.
- This imbalance may signal your immune system, contributing to follicular inflammation and the collapse of tolerance.

Thus, it's not just your immune cells — I, your disturbed microbiome, whisper signals that fan the flames of autoimmunity.

Gut–Skin Axis

The story doesn't end at the scalp. Your **gut microbiome** also influences alopecia areata. Studies suggest that **gut dysbiosis** disrupts immune regulation, priming your body for autoimmune reactions. Remarkably, in a few cases, **faecal microbiota transplantation (FMT)** has led to regrowth of hair — a strong clue that your gut flora and my scalp flora are in dialogue.

Feature	Healthy Scalp Microbiome	Alopecia Areata (Dysbiosis)
Bacterial Balance	Balanced ***Cutibacterium*** and ***Staphylococcus epidermidis*** maintain scalp homeostasis	↑ ***Cutibacterium acnes*** and ↓ ***Staphylococcus epidermidis*** disturb immune tolerance

Feature	Healthy Scalp Microbiome	Alopecia Areata (Dysbiosis)
Fungal Population	***Malassezia restricta*** present in controlled numbers, symbiotic	Imbalance of ***Malassezia species***, contributing to inflammation
Immune Interaction	Hair follicle immune privilege protected, low cytokine activity	**Increased cytokine release** (IFN-γ, IL-15) collapses follicular immune privilege
Follicle Health	Normal cycling, sustained hair growth	**Disrupted cycling**, leading to patchy bald spots
Gut–Skin Link	Stable gut microbiome supports systemic immune balance	**Gut dysbiosis** may worsen scalp inflammation (FMT shows benefit in some cases)

Nutritional & Environmental Influences

Your diet is a major player in hair health. Deficiencies in essential nutrients weaken follicles and worsen alopecia:

- **Iron and zinc** deficiency → impaired hair growth.
- **Niacin and biotin** deficiency → follicular weakening and alopecia.
- **Vitamin D** → critical for hair follicle cycling.
- **Vitamin A** → activates hair follicle stem cells.

In fact, nutritional therapies, especially the **Mediterranean diet** rich in raw vegetables, herbs, and healthy fats or a **high-protein diet**, are being explored to support hair regrowth in alopecia areata patients.

Amazing Facts

1. Alopecia areata is a **non-scarring hair loss**, meaning follicles can regrow if inflammation is controlled.

2. Patients often experience cycles of **hair loss and regrowth**, adding to its unpredictable nature.
3. Stress is a known trigger, influencing immune and microbial balance.
4. Fungal and bacterial imbalances (not just immune cells) are now recognized as important contributors.

Emerging therapies — including **probiotics, postbiotics, and microbiome modulation** — may one day complement immunosuppressants in alopecia management.

Treatment Approaches

1. **Conventional Treatments**
   - **Topical and intralesional corticosteroids** → reduce local immune attack on the hair follicle.
   - **Systemic immunosuppressants** (methotrexate, cyclosporine) → are used in severe cases.
   - **JAK inhibitors (tofacitinib, baricitinib)** → are promising newer therapies that block inflammatory signaling and restore follicle growth.
2. Microbiome-Friendly and Supportive Therapies
   - **Probiotics and prebiotics** → help restore gut microbial balance, which in turn may regulate systemic immunity.
   - **Antifungal balance** → regulating Malassezia populations to avoid excessive scalp inflammation.
   - **Postbiotics (metabolites like short-chain fatty acids)** → under investigation for their immunomodulatory effects.
   - **Dietary correction** → ensuring adequate intake of vitamins A, D, biotin, iron, and zinc.
   - **Mediterranean or high-protein diets** → support follicle health and may reduce relapses.

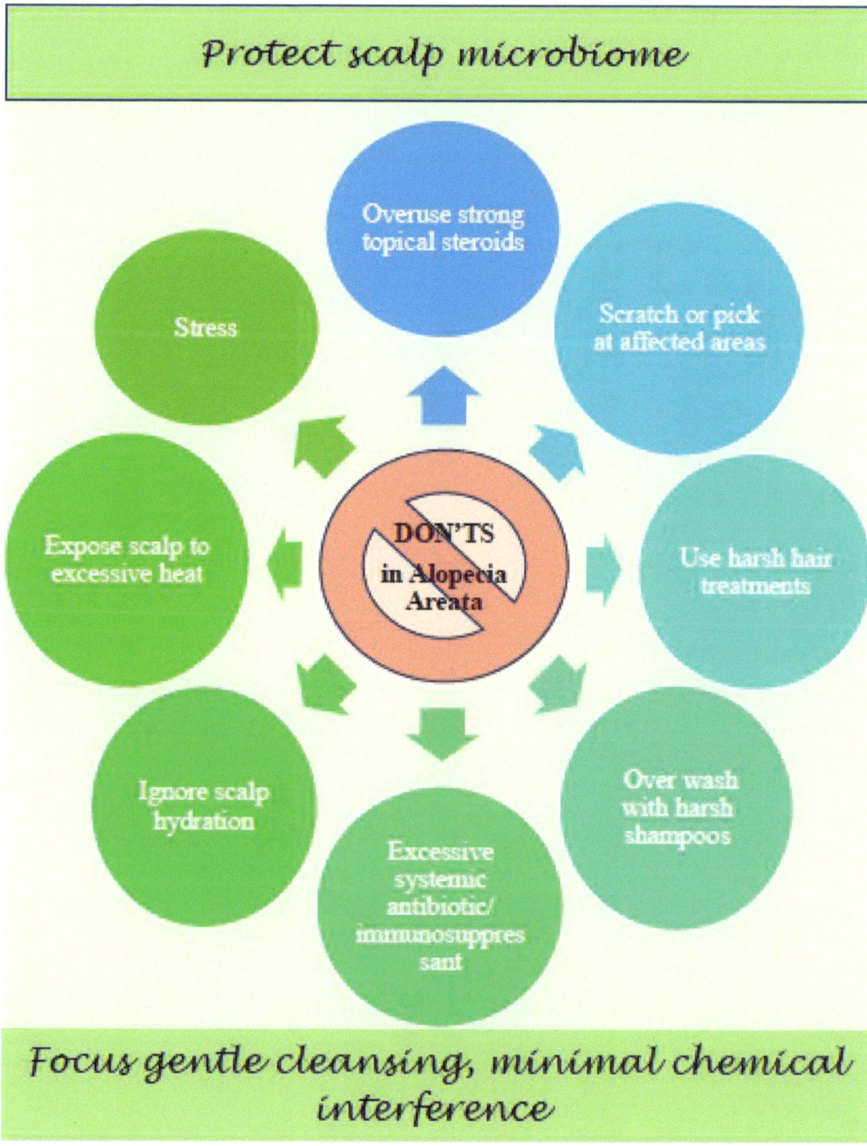

Protect scalp microbiome
Overuse strong topical steroids
Scratch or pick at affected areas
Use harsh hair treatments
Over wash with harsh shampoos
Excessive systemic antibiotic/ immunosuppres sant
Ignore scalp hydration
Expose scalp to excessive heat
Stress
DON'TS in Alopecia Areata
Focus gentle cleansing, minimal chemical interference

"I am your scalp microbiome — usually a quiet guardian of your hair and follicles. When I am balanced, your follicles remain protected, your immune system calm, and your hair grows strong. But when my harmony falters, and your immune system mistakes your follicles for enemies, I cannot shield them. The result is the patchy baldness you call alopecia areata. Care for me with nourishment, balance, and microbial support, and together we may restore the confidence and vitality carried by every strand of your hair."

Chapter 11

Skin Care Products

My Altered Home

"Your skin is a canvas; make sure it's a masterpiece."

My presence on your skin gives you the radiance, texture, and glow you desire. Your skin reflects your inner health and peace. Healthy skin is not an overnight achievement—your skin cells and members of my family, the skin microbiome, are in constant conversation. We discuss, debate, and negotiate; these healthy signals give you that natural radiance. However, environmental exposures throughout your life—including skincare products—can influence the interaction between my microbial family and your skin cells.

The skin microbiome remains relatively stable over the years, but exposures, particularly skincare products, can alter skin chemistry and microbial niches. Understanding relationship between the skin microbiome and skin chemistry is crucial for analysing whether personal habits and product use influence the human skin ecosystem.

The **skin interactome—a novel integration of the genome, microbiome, and exposome—plays a significant role in skin aging and overall skin health.**

The outermost layer of your skin turns over every 3–4 weeks, yet the duration of cosmetic product effects or the persistence of molecules on the skin remains largely unknown. Metabolomic analyses (studies of cellular processes using metabolites produced) reveal correlations between the use of beauty products and variations in the molecular composition of skin. The skin microenvironment, including hormones and pheromones, is dramatically altered by these products.

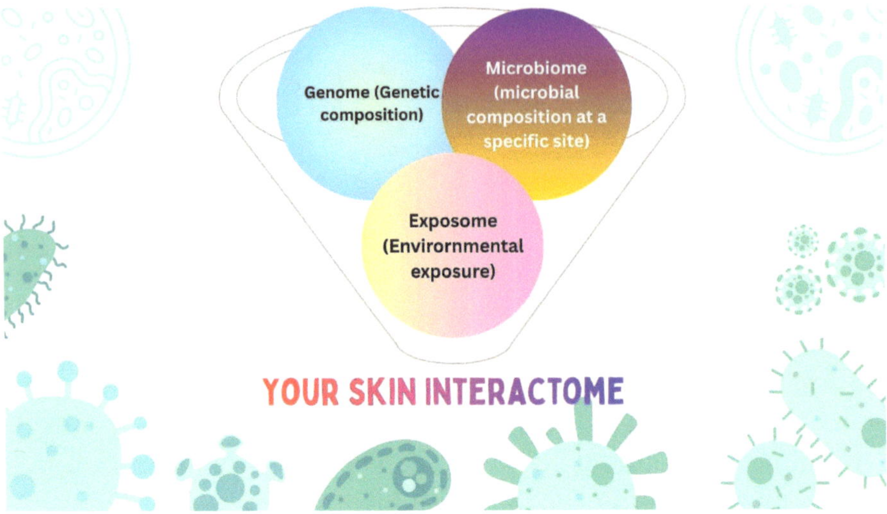

My Voice: How Cosmetics Shape Me, Your Skin Microbiome

I am your **skin microbiome**, helping to maintain your barrier against the outside world. The varied constituents of a skincare regimen can support a healthy microbiome, but some may disrupt it. Imbalances may decrease microbial diversity, hinder the growth of beneficial microbes, and increase susceptibility to infections. Cosmetics, intended for cleansing or beautification, introduce a broad range of chemicals that interact with my home, potentially causing alterations.

> The long term effects of these products is potentially not conductive to 'good skin'. In addition, skin care products are designed to provide colour, glow, healthiness, or to treat blemishes and cuts and/or infections have an indirect or direct impact on transient as well as resident microbial skin flora.

Every cosmetic product you apply touches me first—and can either strengthen or weaken me.

Let me tell you how.

Skin products can be alcohol- or oil-based, often containing complex ingredients. They may provide color, glow, or treat blemishes and infections, indirectly or directly impacting both resident and transient skin microbes. Alcohols and salicylic acid, for instance, may act as nonselective surface killers, altering microbial communities over time. Daily cleansing can strip microorganisms from the skin, yet the skin microbiome is surprisingly resilient and often rebounds after short-term disruptions. However, frequent or long-term use can make it harder for the microbiome to regain its natural balance.

1. **Moisturizers: Feeding My Lipophilic Members**
   When you apply moisturizers rich in lipids, I receive new nutrients. My **lipophilic members**—like *Staphylococcus* and *Cutibacterium (Propionibacterium) acnes*—feed on these lipid components. Sometimes, they grow excessively, tipping my balance. This overgrowth can disturb microbial diversity and increase the risk of skin conditions. Moderation in lipid-rich formulations helps prevent one group from dominating at the expense of others.

2. **Preservatives: The Silent but Persistent Disturbers**
   Preservatives are designed to protect your products, but they rarely spare me. Compounds such as **parabens, phenoxyethanol, and 1,2-hexanediol** kill not just pathogens, but also my beneficial commensals like *Staphylococcus epidermidis* and *Cutibacterium acnes*. Evidence shows that **commensal bacteria are often more sensitive to preservatives than pathogens**, which leaves me vulnerable to colonization by harmful species. Worse still, preservatives remain biologically active long after application, continuing to influence me. Their long-term ecological effects on my communities are still poorly understood, but I can already feel their pressure every day.

3. **Cleansers: pH and Surfactants as Double-Edged Swords**
   I flourish best at an acidic pH of about 5.0, but many cleansers raise this to 7–8. A more alkaline environment disrupts my equilibrium, suppressing beneficial bacteria and inviting opportunists. **Harsh surfactants** damage the lipid bilayers of your **stratum corneum**, increasing **transepidermal water loss (TEWL)** and causing dehydration. Cleansers containing **NaOH** can promote fungal overgrowth, such as *Candida spp.*, which are opportunistic pathogens. Added allergens, irritants, or even microplastics further stress both your skin and me, increasing the risk of **allergic contact dermatitis**.

When Cosmetic Compounds Help Me

Not every chemical harms me. Some actives in skincare regulate the growth of harmful microbes such as *Staphylococcus aureus* or acne-associated *C. acnes*. They can block biofilm formation and restore microbial equilibrium. In controlled amounts, these compounds act as allies. But when you overuse them, even my commensals suffer. The lesson is clear: balance in exposure is critical for me to stay resilient.

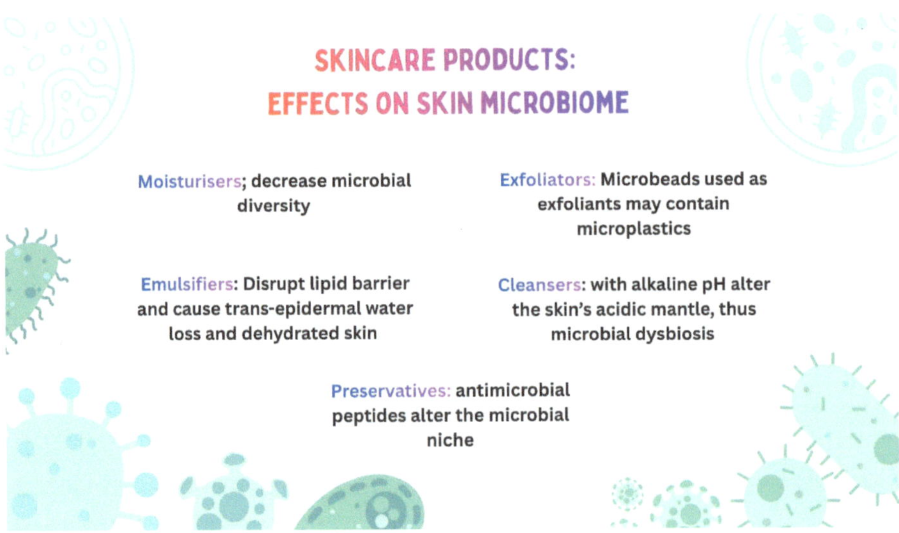

New Frontiers: Microbiome-Friendly Innovations

Fortunately, the future is brighter. Cosmetic scientists are creating formulations with me in mind.

- **Preservative-free and low-pH products** allow my diversity to expand. For instance, **native algae masks** maintain low skin pH, suppressing harmful *Corynebacterium* while sustaining overall microbial richness.
- **Natural antioxidants**, such as **dragon fruit (*Hylocereus undatus*) extract**, support me by reducing oxidative stress and fostering microbial stability.
- **Prebiotics, probiotics, and postbiotics** are powerful allies. Prebiotics nourish my beneficial members, probiotics introduce supportive strains, and postbiotics provide microbial metabolites that help me regulate your barrier. These approaches prevent dysbiosis and encourage homeostasis.

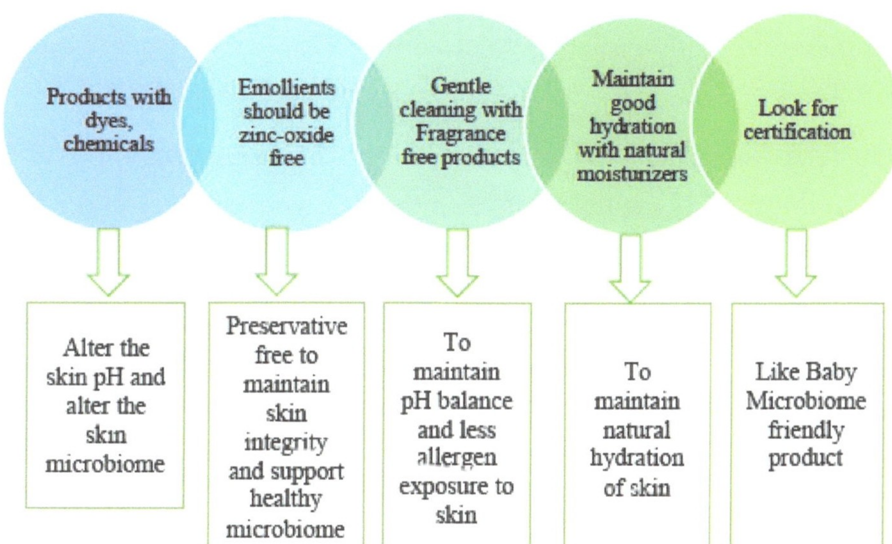

Special Care for Baby Skin

When you were an infant, I was only beginning to establish myself. Early microbial colonization shapes lifelong skin and immune health. Baby products with harsh chemicals can damage this foundation irreversibly. But **gentle, microbiome-friendly ingredients**—such as **inulin, rhamnose, and glucomannan**—help me grow in harmony, ensuring a protective and balanced start for your life.

What I Do for You Every Day

Never forget, I am not passive. I actively work to keep you healthy:

- My **proteases** restore your stratum corneum after damage.
- My **lipases** recycle sebum lipids, stabilizing hydration and indirectly influencing TEWL.
- My **ureases** regulate urea breakdown, preventing dehydration.
- I produce **bacteriocins** to suppress pathogens.
- I form **biofilms** to strengthen microbial resilience.
- Through **quorum sensing**, I coordinate microbial communication.
- I maintain your **acidic pH shield**, crucial for barrier integrity and defense.

My Allies: Probiotics, Prebiotics, and Synbiotics

When disruption occurs, I can recover—but your choices make the process easier. Proper diet, stress removal, and the use of probiotics, prebiotics, and synbiotics can promote my regrowth. Prebiotics—nutrients that selectively feed my beneficial members—further enrich my protective families, while synbiotics combine both approaches to maximize skin health. Even topical bacterial extracts are being tested to see how they reinforce my commensal balance.

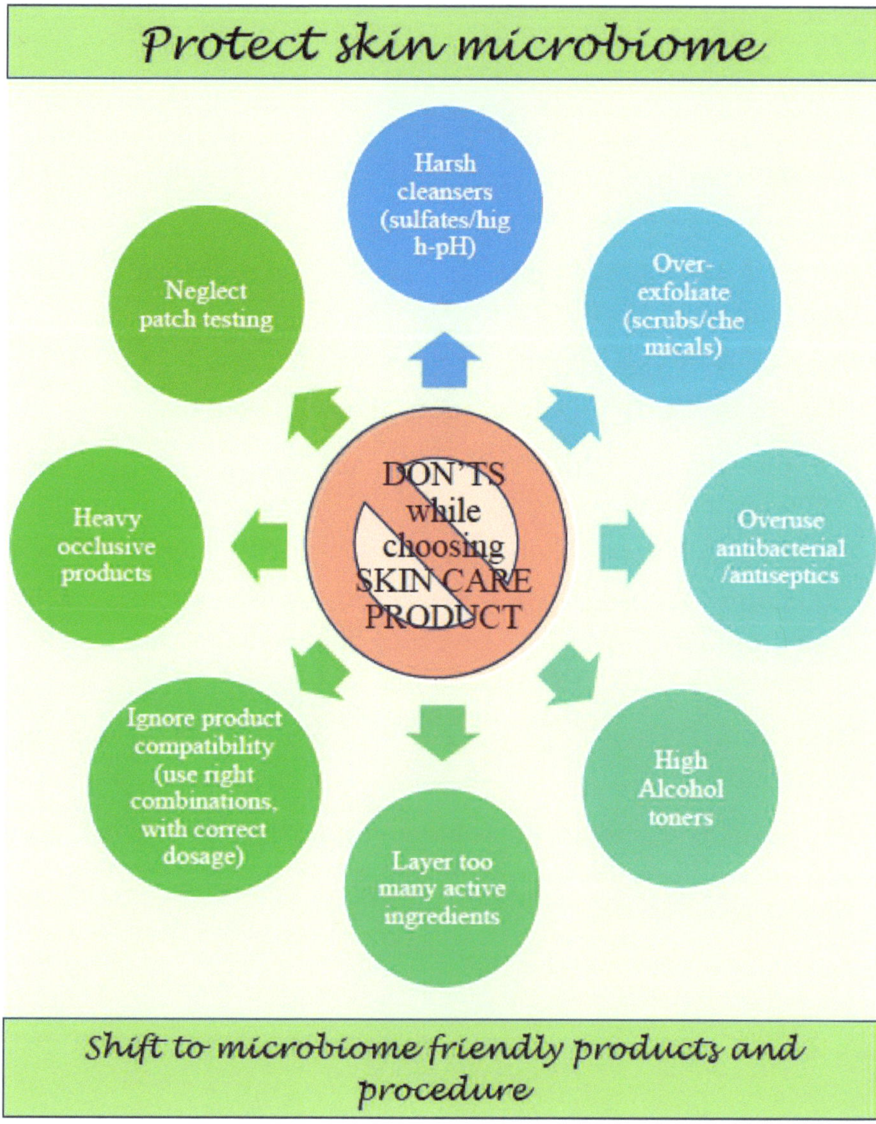
Protect skin microbiome
Harsh cleansers (sulfates/high-pH)
Over-exfoliate (scrubs/chemicals)
Overuse antibacterial /antiseptics
High Alcohol toners
Layer too many active ingredients
Ignore product compatibility (use right combinations, with correct dosage)
Heavy occlusive products
Neglect patch testing
DON'TS while choosing SKIN CARE PRODUCT
Shift to microbiome friendly products and procedure

Key message

1. Cosmetics are not neutral—they are active partners in shaping me.
2. Microbiome changes may be transient (stressors like washing or alcohol-based products), but generally return to baseline, reflecting the resilience of skin flora.
3. Frequent or prolonged use can make recovery difficult, causing long-term shifts.
4. **Preservatives and alkaline cleansers** can weaken me, reducing diversity and stripping away protective commensals.
    - Preservatives with antimicrobial properties (parabens, 1,2-hexanediol, phenoxyethanol) can inhibit resident *Staphylococcus epidermidis* and *Cutibacterium acnes.*
    - Alkaline cleansers (pH 7–8) disturb the skin's natural acidic environment (pH ~5), favoring pathogenic microbes and increasing TEWL (trans-epidermal water loss).
5. **Overuse of actives** can silence my allies while encouraging opportunists.
6. But when you choose **microbiome-friendly, low-pH, balanced, and natural formulations**, you empower me to protect you.

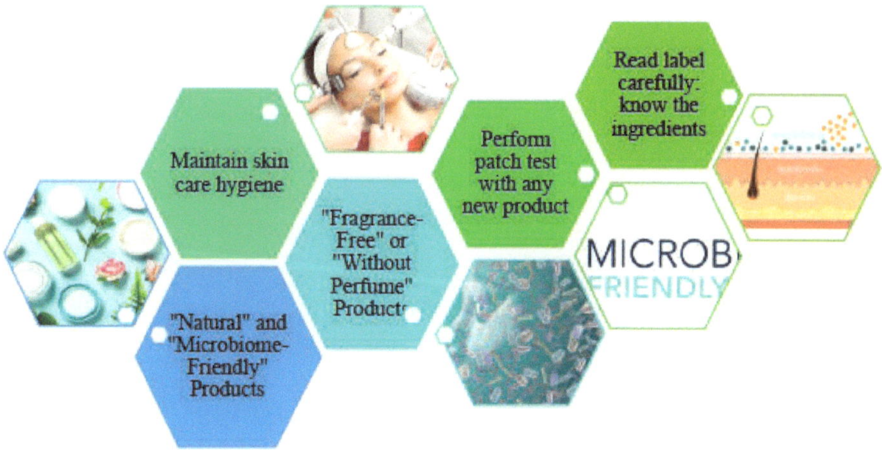

"I am your first line of defence. When you care for me, I care for you—with resilience, protection, and radiant skin health. Together, we are stronger."

Chapter 12

Skin Microbiome Restoration

Restoring My Happy Home with Pre-, Pro-, and Synbiotics

I, your **skin microbiome**, am your microscopic family living on every inch of your skin. My home is your skin, and just like any community, we thrive when balance is maintained. But sometimes, this balance is disrupted—through genetics, environmental stress, diet, or aging—and that's when skin conditions appear. Acne, eczema, psoriasis, dryness, and even wrinkles? Those are signals that our harmony is disturbed.

As already mentioned, I don't live in isolation. I am constantly communicating with your **gut microbiome** through what scientists call the **gut-skin axis**. Metabolites, microbial signals, and immune messages travel through your bloodstream, influencing how I function, how your immune system responds, and how healthy your skin looks. When this communication breaks down, it's not just your gut that suffers—your skin shows it too.

Thus, it is important to have a balanced home to provide you a resilient skin.

How You Can Help Me Thrive

The beneficial effect of nutribiotics/pharmabiotics on skin can be achieved by:

Ingesting/ Topical applications-

- Beneficial microorganisms
- Nutrients for good microbes
- Beneficial metabolic products of healthy microbes

I love **food**—but not just any food. I thrive on **prebiotics**, enjoy the company of **probiotics**, and benefit from the byproducts of microbial metabolism called **postbiotics**. Together, they form **synbiotics**, a power combo that helps me restore balance and make your skin glow.

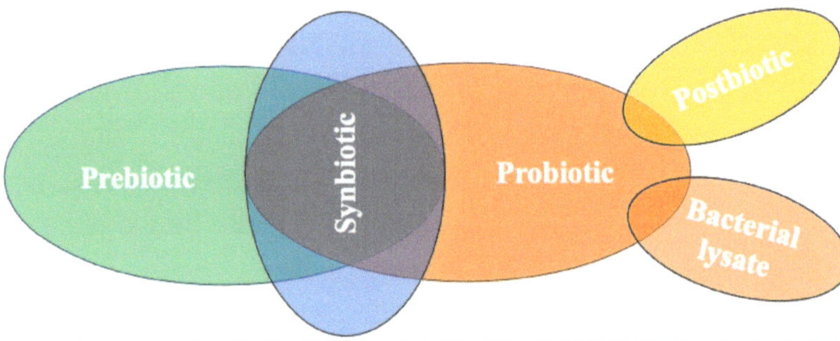

Beneficial forms of microbes delivered in topical/oral formulations

Prebiotics- Compounds that foster growth or activity of beneficial microorganisms.

Probiotics- Friendly microbes, with beneficial effect on human body.

Postbiotics- Bioactive compounds as biogenics, or simply metabolites; are soluble factors, secreted by beneficial microbes, or released after microbial lysis providing physiological benefits to the host

Synbiotics - Combination of probiotics and prebiotics, essentially a synergistic mixture intended to enhance the survival, implantation, and beneficial effects of probiotics. **Bacterial extract/bacterial lysate -** A substance derived from bacteria, containing various components like proteins, metabolites, or cell wall materials, used with proven beneficial impact of human health.

A number of products containing prebiotics, probiotics or synbiotics are marketed as commercial topical skin care products. Topical and oral formulations of prebiotics and postbiotics are becoming an essential part of skin care regimens across the world. Interestingly, due to the evident gut-skin axis, nutritional products containing prebiotics and/or probiotics have a positive effect on skin by modulating the immune system and by providing therapeutic benefits for various skin diseases, such as acne vulgaris, atopic dermatitis, and psoriasis.

Topical and oral formulations containing bacterial extracts, prebiotics, postbiotics and synbiotics have been demonstrated to have a beneficial impact on skin health.

Topical probiotic/topical prebiotic	**Oral probiotics/prebiotics**
Nourish the beneficial microbiomes	Increase the diversity of gut microbiota
Maintain epithelial barrier	Enhance immune function
Fighting pathogens, promoting overall balance in the skin microbiome	Improve digestion- maintain gut motility
Regulate moisture, thus maintain hydration	Help synthesis of essential vitamins
Regulate sebum production	Maintain intestinal homeostasis

Prebiotics: The Feast for My Friendly Residents

The term prebiotic was developed initially to describe materials (carbohydrates) that travel to the colon when ingested and there in promote the growth of desirable (probiotic) organisms.

In cosmetic formulations, the term prebiotic can be applied ‘in principle’ to the skin microbiota where the carbohydrates stimulate selectively the activity and growth of beneficial ‘normal’ skin microbiota.

'**Prebiotics**' are defined as **'a selectively fermented ingredient that allows specific changes**, both in the composition and/or activity in the microflora that confers benefits upon host well-being and health'. **When you eat or apply prebiotics, it's like supplying me with the right nutrients to thrive and defend your skin.**

Prebiotics are **selectively fermented compounds** that feed the good microbes among us. Think of oligosaccharides, inulin, sorbitol, raffinose, konjac glucomannan—they are like gourmet meals for the helpful members of my community.

The main prebiotics used in cosmetic products are konjac glucomannan, fructooligosaccharide, glucomannan.

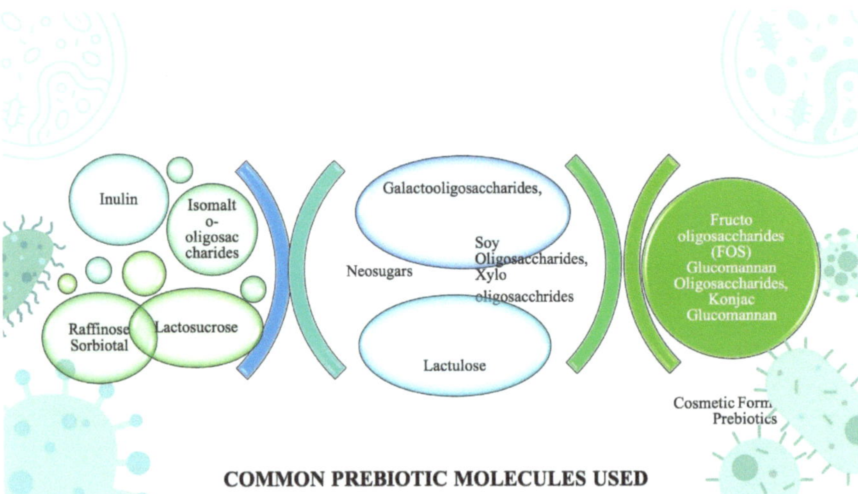

- When you apply prebiotics or ingest them, I can **grow faster than the pathogens**, that often cause acne and flare-ups.
- Prebiotics help me **communicate with your immune system**, encouraging anti-inflammatory responses, which calm irritated skin.
- Prebiotics regulate **sebum production**, keeping pores clear and preventing acne formation.

- Konjac glucomannan hydrolysates have been shown to exert a positive and direct impact on skin health:
  - Unblocking the pores on the skin surface and restoring skin barrier properties and controling superficial microbiota.
  - Reducing acne vulgaris and inducing a glow to the skin.
  - Modulating skin bacterial proliferation and normalizing sensitive skin barrier functionality.
  - Having a positive effect to prevent atopic diseases.
  - Reducing eczema severity in children
- Glucooligosaccharides, can control the growth of *S. aureus*, which often infects or colonises patients with atopic dermatitis .

Probiotics: New Friends in My Neighbourhood

Probiotics, 'live microorganisms' that, when administered in adequate amounts, confer health benefits on the host'.

Probiotics are **live microorganisms** that come to live among me. When you introduce them through your diet or topicals, we team up to protect your skin. My favorite strains include *Lactobacillus plantarum, Lactobacillus rhamnosus, Lactobacillus reuteri,* and *Bifidobacterium longum.*

Here's what we do together:

- **Occupy my spaces** so that harmful microbes don't settle in.
- **Produce antimicrobial compounds** (like bacteriocins and acids) that directly fight pathogens.
- **Train your immune cells** to respond appropriately, reducing inflammation and calming flare-ups.
- **Neutralize free radicals**, protecting your skin from UV damage and aging.

Probiotics have the capacity to optimise, maintain and restore the microbiota of the skin in different ways.

Probiotics continuously trigger the skin natural defences:

i. By competition with pathogens for nutrients
ii. Contesting for mucosal adherence sites
iii. Modulating the mucosal immune function
iv. Production of antimicrobial metabolites like bacteriocins to regulate growth of other microbes
v. Restore the balance between free radical scavengers and free radical production.
vi. combination of probiotics and prebiotics can benefit skin conditions by increasing skin hydration and decreasing phenol production levels

Probiotics, such as *Lactobacillus* and *Bifidobacterium*, are now recognized as nutricosmetic agents. They help me counteract oxidative stress, maintain pH balance, and repair barrier dysfunction.

- *Bifidobacterium breve, Lactobacillus plantarum,* and *Lactobacillus reuteri* reduce UV-induced photoaging and improve hydration.
- Exopolysaccharides (EPS) from *Lactobacillus plantarum HY7714* show antioxidant and immunomodulatory activity, boosting my resilience.

We've been studied extensively: *Lactobacillus rhamnosus* GG, for instance, can prevent eczema in infants; topical *Vitreoscilla filiformis* reduces *S. aureus* and inflammation in atopic dermatitis. Together, we restore order when chaos tries to take over your skin.

Postbiotics: Gifts Left Behind by Our Friends

Sometimes, even after probiotics leave, their **metabolites** remain—and we benefit greatly from them. These are called postbiotics.

Short-chain fatty acids (SCFAs), exopolysaccharides (EPS), and bioactive peptides **help me**:

- **Strengthen the barrier** by improving tight junctions in your skin.
- **Reduce inflammation** and oxidative stress.
- **Support collagen production**, keeping your skin elastic and smooth.

Clinical studies confirm that postbiotic creams lower **trans epidermal water loss**, restore hydration, and reduce sensitivity. They are like tiny repair kits, left behind by our helpful microbial neighbours.

Synbiotics: The Ultimate Teamwork

When prebiotics and probiotics come together, we call them **synbiotics**. It's like hosting a neighbourhood festival: prebiotics feed the probiotics, probiotics keep the pathogens in check, and together, we create an environment where everyone thrives.

> The main purpose of synbiotic is addition of substrates (i.e prebiotics) to increase the increase the survival of the probiotic strains. Synbiotics have the capacity to optimise, maintain and restore the microbiota of the skin systemically or by topical applications.

Here's how synbiotics work:

- Boost our survival and colonization on your skin
- Enhance systemic and local immune responses

- Improve hydration, barrier function, and resilience against environmental stress

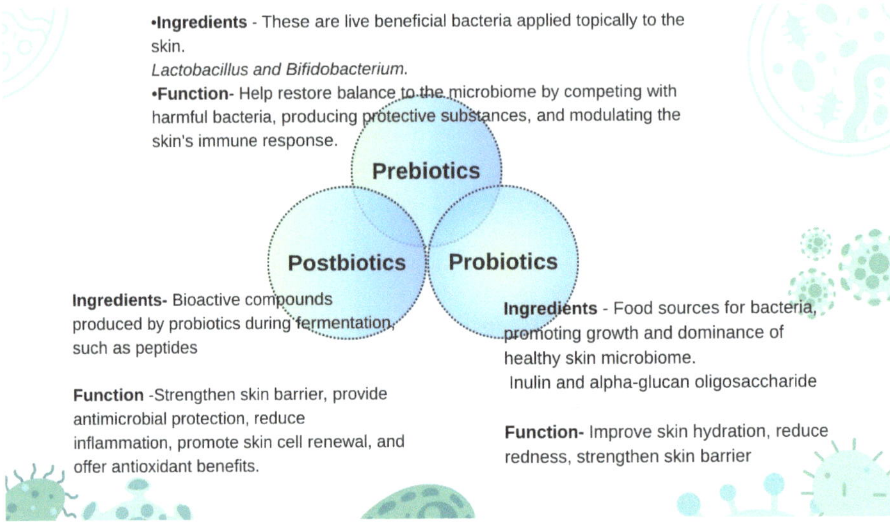

My Friends from Within: How Gut Microbes Help Your Skin

My distant relatives living in your gut, not just keeping your digestion in check—they communicate with me too. This gut-skin connection explains why certain skin conditions sometimes start in your digestive system. An unhealthy gut—what scientists call microbial dysbiosis—increases intestinal permeability, which can lead to:

- Accumulation of bacterial metabolites in your skin
- Impairment of epidermal differentiation and skin integrity

Thankfully, your gut friends—prebiotics, probiotics, and postbiotics—help restore harmony.

They normalize gut flora, prevent chronic inflammation, and even enhance adaptive immune responses, especially important as we get older.

When you take oral probiotics, they don't just stay in the gut—they help me directly:

- Reduce visible signs of skqaain aging
- Normalize the skin's acidic pH
- Combat oxidative stress and damage from sunlight
- Enhance your skin barrier function, keeping me strong and resilient

So remember, I'm not working alone. Treat your gut well, and I thrive, helping your skin stay healthy, balanced, and glowing from the inside out.

Major challenges in developing probiotic and synbiotic topical formulations with beneficial results include:

i. Maintaining the viability of probiotic microbes in the formulation (prebiotics are retained even in relatively harsh formats).

ii. Ability of the good bacteria to recolonise the skin after application (harsh environmental conditions of the skin preventing colonisation of probiotic microbes)

iii. Harsh preservatives or surfactants in cosmetic products can kill both harmful and helpful microbes

iv. Environmental stress (UV, pollution, humidity): continuous environmental exposure disrupts my balance

v. Poor hygiene or inconsistent skincare : body hygiene practices of the individual and constant association of topical application with clothing.

Final Words from Your Skin Microbiome

I am always changing, reacting to your diet, lifestyle, environment, and age. My health is directly linked to yours. When we are balanced:

- Your skin glows and feels smooth
- Inflammation and sensitivity are reduced
- Signs of aging are delayed

"By feeding me well—with prebiotics, probiotics, postbiotics, and synbiotics—you support your skin from the inside out and from the outside in. A diverse and balanced microbiome is not just my home—it's the secret to your healthy, youthful, resilient skin."